Where are the Gaps?

HIV and Gender Pre-service Teacher Training Curriculum and Practices in East Africa

Iffat Farah, Caroline Kavuma,
Mweru Mwingi and Orwe Onyango

COMMONWEALTH SECRETARIAT

Commonwealth Secretariat
Marlborough House, Pall Mall
London SW1Y 5HX
United Kingdom

Published by the Commonwealth Secretariat
Edited by editors4change Limited
Cover design by Tattersall Hammarling & Silk
Printed by RPM Print & Design

Cover photo: Jenny Matthews/Panos Pictures

Copies of this publication may be obtained from

The Publications Section
Commonwealth Secretariat
Marlborough House, Pall Mall
London SW1Y 5HX
United Kingdom
Tel: +44 (0)20 7747 6534
Fax: +44 (0)20 7839 9081
Email: publications@commonwealth.int
Web: www.thecommonwealth.org/publications

A catalogue record for this publication is available from the British Library.

ISBN: 978-1-84929-001-2 (paperback)
ISBN: 978-1-84859-034-2 (downloadable e-book)

About the Authors

The authors are affiliated with The Aga Khan University, Institute for Educational Development, East Africa.

Acknowledgements

First of all, we would like to thank the Ministries of Education in Kenya, Tanzania and Uganda for giving us permission to undertake this review and access teacher education institutions in their respective countries, and for taking the time to participate in the consultative workshop. We are also thankful to the various education departments for sharing curriculum documents and other relevant information with us.

A number of people helped us collect information about curriculum implementation in colleges. We would like to acknowledge and thank the following: Naureen Madhani, Head of Administration, Aga Khan University, Institute for Educational Development, Eastern Africa; Ibrahim Nandwa, Professional Development Tutor, Aga Khan High School, Mombasa; Charles Osore, Professional Development Tutor, Aga Khan High School, Mombasa; Charles Maina, Professional Development Tutor, St Charles Lwanga; Alice Mugoya Ibale, Programme Manager, PIASCY Project; George Opiro, Commissioner, Guidance and Counselling, MOES, Uganda; Issa Bakari, Education Officer, Ministry of Education and Vocational Development, Tanzania; and Khamis Mmanga, Professional Development Tutor, Nkrumah Teacher Training College, Zanzibar.

Our special thanks go to the principals, tutors and students of the colleges who participated in this study. This review would not be possible without their co-operation and their generosity in giving us their time.

Naureen Madhani, Sarah Ojuando and Ubaldus Tumaini, AKU-IED, East Africa, helped in finding information on HIV prevalence. Sarah also helped with organising and formatting the report. Thank you to all.

Finally, we would like to thank the Commonwealth Secretariat who funded the review. We are particularly grateful to Dr Jyotsna Jha who provided support throughout the period of conducting this review.

Contents

Foreword vii

List of Abbreviations x

1. Introduction 1

2. Review Methodology 6

3. The Context 8

4. Structure and Scope of School Education in East Africa 10

5. Structure and Scope of Pre-service Teacher Education in East Africa 15

6. The Policy Context for HIV and Gender Education 17

7. Teacher Education Curriculum 20

8. Curriculum in Practice 68

9. Gaps Between Policy, Curriculum and Practice Across the Three Countries 89

10. Recommendations 91

Appendix: HIV and AIDS and Gender Study Dissemination Workshop, 11–13 March 2008 93

References 97

Tables

3.1 Estimated number of people (adults and children) living with HIV 8

3.2 Estimated rate of HIV and AIDS prevalence among young men and women (2007 figures) 9

4.1 Education in East Africa 10
5.1 Teacher training and certification in Kenya, Uganda and Tanzania 16
7.1 Organisation of the primary teacher education (PTE) syllabus in Kenya 21
7.2 Carrier subjects and integrated HIV content in the 2004 primary teacher education (PTE) syllabus in Kenya 23
7.3 Number of teachers trained through different teacher education programmes in Tanzania 33
7.4 Analysis of the certificate course in teacher education 34
7.5 Analysis of the diploma course in teacher education 39
7.6 Integration of HIV and gender into the subject syllabus in primary teacher education curriculum in Uganda 46
7.7 Integration of HIV and gender into teacher education courses at university in Uganda 56
7.8 HIV and gender material used in primary teacher education in Uganda 64

Foreword

HIV and AIDS has emerged as a major threat in many countries to the educational gains achieved over the last decades. The worst affected region is sub-Saharan Africa, and this includes a number of Commonwealth countries. More than 113 million children in the world are estimated to be affected by HIV through loss of one or both parents, increased family responsibilities or through illness themselves. In Zambia and Kenya, for example, it is projected that there will be 2 to 3 million AIDS orphans by 2010. Girls particularly are at risk, with two-thirds of all children currently affected being girls. Girls and women also share disproportionate responsibility of care. However, it is important to note that girls and women are also more adversely affected by HIV in Africa and elsewhere simply because they have a secondary status in society.

Although the impact of HIV on education systems can be far reaching, the role that education itself can play in effective protection against the epidemic is crucial. Education can promote awareness and support behaviour change, both with regard to HIV and issues of gender. Research, however, suggests that the potential impact of education is not being realised. Deep rooted values and social practices are resistant to change. Awareness generation is important, but it can only serve as a first step in changing behaviour.

Teachers can play an important role in changing attitudes and behaviour, particularly in developing contexts. Yet, a Commonwealth Association for the Development of Education in Africa (ADEA) Africa regional workshop, Identifying Good Practices in the Education Sector's Response to HIV and AIDS, held in 2006, identified that insufficient teacher preparation was leading to ineffective communication of key messages to students, parents and their communities. This was particularly so with regard to addressing issues of social/religious taboo and discrimination. Limitations in the delivery of effective and empowering gender education were also seen as a major challenge. The workshop findings expressed the need for strengthening of teacher preparation practices, but it was recognised that greater understanding of the current teacher education curriculum and practices was required in order to determine how to challenge and alter behaviour. Following on from the workshop, a review of teacher education curriculum and practices was therefore initiated. The selected countries were three East African countries: Kenya, Tanzania and Uganda, where the rate of HIV and AIDS is high and where girls continue to face disparity in various ways.

The review sought therefore to consider not only the policies and curriculum, but also the ways in which these are translated into practices. Drawing on a comprehensive desk review of relevant materials, and in-depth interviews of tutors and trainee teachers, the report concludes that although the three countries have a strong and encouraging policy context mandating the inclusion of HIV and AIDS education in the school curricula and by extension into teacher training, the gap between policy and implementation is wide. The objectives and the content on HIV and gender aim only at providing factual knowledge and to raise awareness among teachers. They do not reflect the aim of preparing future teachers to teach children and young adults to change their behaviour. Little attention is given to engage trainees to examine their existing beliefs, attitudes and behaviour, or to learn how to teach these topics to children in schools. Where gender topics are included, they represent a reinforcement of current gender roles and relationships, or take a welfare approach rather than strengthening women's agency, necessary for their well-being. Gender finds even less space than HIV in the curricula and in the teaching.

As well as systematically examining the gaps between curriculum, syllabus and practices, the report also highlights weaknesses in tutor preparation in teacher training institutions. It suggests that tutors' own beliefs and attitudes can act as a major constraint and it considers ways of addressing this issue.

Following on from the findings of the study, a pilot Action project, led by the Aga Khan University, Institute for Educational Development: Eastern Africa, Dar es Salaam, Tanzania (AKU: IED) and in collaboration with a number of Tanzanian teacher training institutions, has been initiated. Its objective is to take the lessons learned in order to actively improve the content and methodology of teaching HIV and AIDS in the colleges that participated in the curriculum review. It is also intended that the experience gained will support the development of a framework for action in other institutions and countries. The experiences will provide the basis for a guide towards the improvement of the teaching of HIV-related topics in teacher training institutions and in turn in schools.

We hope that whatever your role, teacher, student, academic, government officer, representative of a development agency or an interested individual, you will find this publication both of interest and practical use.

Caroline Pontefract
Director, Social Transformation Programmes Division (STPD)
Commonwealth Secretariat
London, UK

January 2009

List of Abbreviations

ADEA	Association for the Development of Education in Africa
AIDS	Acquired immune deficiency syndrome
AKU:IED	Aga Khan University, Institute for Educational Development
BEd	Bachelor of Education
BTE	Bachelor of Teacher Education
CASE	Certificate of Advanced Secondary Education
CfBT	Centre for British Teachers
CSE	Certificate of Secondary Education
ECD	Early childhood development
ECED	Early childhood education development
EFA	Education For All
GER	Gross enrolment ratio
HDI	Human Development Index
HIV	Human immunodeficiency virus
ICT	Information and communication technology
KCSE	Kenya Certificate of Secondary Education
MGSC&SS	Ministry of Gender, Sports, Culture and Social Services (Kenya)
MOES	Ministry of Education and Sports (Uganda)
MOEST	Ministry of Education, Science and Technology (Kenya)
NER	Net enrolment ratio
NGO	Non-governmental organisation
NTC	National Training College
PIASCY	Presidential Initiative on the AIDS Strategy for Communication to Youth
PLWA	People living with AIDS
PSABH	Primary School Action for Better Health
PTC	Primary teachers' college
PTE	Primary teacher education
ROK	Republic of Kenya
STD	Sexually transmitted disease
STI	Sexually transmitted infection

TBA	Traditional birth attendant
TIE	Tanzania Institute of Education
TTC	Teacher Training College
UACE	Uganda Advanced Certificate of Education
UCE	Uganda Certificate of Education
UNAIDS	Joint UN Programme on HIV/AIDS
UNESCO	United Nations Educational, Scientific and Cultural Organization
UNICEF	UN Children's Fund
UPE	Universal primary education
VCT	Voluntary counselling and testing
WHO	World Health Organization

Chapter 1

Introduction

'*Among health concerns, infectious diseases are having a devastating impact on school systems worldwide. …The situation is particularly critical in sub-Saharan Africa, which accounts for 63 per cent of the global HIV-infected population, 89 per cent of malaria-related deaths, and 12 of the 15 countries with the highest tuberculosis incidence rate worldwide …). Women increasingly carry the burden of HIV and AIDS, either through infection or as caretakers*' (UNESCO, 2007b).

The school systems in sub-Saharan Africa have been severely affected by HIV and AIDS.[1] The effects include:

- very high rates of infection and death among teachers, thus reducing the available workforce;
- high absenteeism among teachers, who are themselves infected or who have to take care of infected others;
- an increase in the number of orphan children;
- an increase in absenteeism among students, who have to become caretakers of ill parents or siblings due to loss of parents; and to
- HIV and social and emotional problems among such children.

Education, especially girls' education, is seen as the most effective protection against the HIV epidemic, and as a way of raising awareness about health, sanitation and nutrition. Hargreaves and Boler (2006) reviewed findings from research carried out between 1990 and 2006 and concluded that education enables girls to have better control over their sexual behaviour, and that girls with secondary education have a lower risk of HIV as compared with those who have no or only primary school education. Other studies suggest that providing HIV prevention programmes at primary school are more successful in positively influencing sexual behaviour (Gallant and Maticka-Tyandale, 2003; cited in Clarke, 2005).

While there is plenty of evidence to support the very significant role of education on reducing the risk of being infected and on a person's ability to cope with the disease, there is also evidence that the education systems in general have not been very successful in fulfilling this role. Based on research with young people in Tanzania, Vavrus (2003) argues that general education per se cannot always protect against HIV. Targeted and specific information about HIV and AIDS, as part of a robust curriculum, is needed for any significant impact from the years of education. Other research studies also suggest that 'effective' HIV education in schools can have a positive impact on the sexual behaviour of young people (James-Traore, Finger, Ruland and Savariaud, 2004).

Gender is a cross-cutting issue in education. Gender equality in education in a broad sense means creating equal opportunities for both boys and girls, so that in all respects they can access education, participate and learn equally. We also know that girls in most societies continue to be disadvantaged and still constitute about two-thirds of all the world's out-of-school children in the primary school age group. A majority of the young people estimated to be infected and affected by HIV and AIDS in sub-Saharan Africa are female. In 2004, among the age group 15–24, the overall ratio of infection female to male was 2:1. This ratio for sub-Saharan Africa was 3:1 (UNICEF, 2004).

Girls and women are more likely to be infected and affected because of the cultural and socio-economic contexts in which they live. Women have limited power to negotiate safe sex and often suffer from male violence. Poverty among women is high and they have limited access to paid jobs outside the home. This poverty may lead them to engage in sex for money or material goods. Girls' participation in school is adversely affected by their own and their families' poor health status. They are expected to take on the role as caregivers, which can keep them from attending school. Girls' experience of schooling is also negatively affected by sexual harassment in schools and teenage pregnancy.

Education processes in schools are not necessarily gender responsive and the role of teachers in addressing gender issues and HIV remains minimal. Clarke (2005) shows that gender analysis and gender issues are often missing in HIV education policy and programmes, and argues that an effective education response to HIV requires both mainstreaming of gender and HIV into policy, curriculum and practice. Schools and teachers are currently unprepared to respond to the gendered needs of their pupils in the context of HIV. For example, a study conducted in Uganda (Kakuru, 2007, shows that female students and teachers are more affected by HIV and AIDS, yet ... '*teachers are required to treat boys and girls equally. They cannot take into account the impact of HIV and AIDS on pupils in their classroom management strategies. They expect all children to turn up on time for example, with all necessary supplies, regardless of their circumstances*'.

According to UNESCO (2006), the ultimate goal of HIV and AIDS education is to enable learners to adopt protective behaviour for their health and wellbeing, and to show respect to and concern for others. The components necessary to meet these goals would include basic knowledge on: health, sexuality and HIV; human rights and stigma; relationships and gender issues; and life skills, such as critical thinking, problem solving and decision-making, necessary for promotion of physical and mental wellbeing. It is also important that the school is gender sensitive, does not encourage gender bias and gender stereotyping and that there is a curriculum which includes content and practices to promote gender equality in and outside the class (UNESCO, 2006).

Education sector responses to HIV and gender issues have varied. However, most countries in Africa have formulated HIV and gender-specific policies and strategies, and have prepared HIV strategic plans for the education sector (Rispel, Letlape and Metcalf, 2006). In several countries, HIV has been included in the primary and secondary school curricula and in prepared teaching/learning materials. However, evidence about the implementation and impact of this initiative is not unanimously positive (UNESCO, 2007a).

There is some evidence to suggest that the '*quality of the implementation* [of curricula] *is probably more important than the detailed design of materials or curricula*', and that good quality teacher training and support are critical in implementing curricula for effective HIV education in schools (James-Traore, Finger, Ruland and Savariaud, 2004). There is a growing body of research that suggests teacher quality is the main determinant of students' outcomes. For example, Darling-Hammond (2000) notes that teacher quality is one of the most important factors contributing to student achievement, more significant than class size (National Institute of Education, 2008).

The importance of teacher quality for effective HIV and AIDS education in schools is also being recognised. A review of AIDS and teacher training in ten African countries (UNESCO, 2006) underscores the importance of teachers for effective HIV education, and calls for strategies to minimise the impact of HIV on teachers and to maximise teachers' contributions to the fight against this pandemic. The Education for All (EFA) monitoring report (2008) emphasises the same point when it concludes that '*Introduction of HIV and AIDS education in the curriculum needs to be complemented by professional development of teachers*' (UNESCO, 2007a, p.132).

Thus, successful implementation of an HIV and gender education curriculum would depend the ability of the teachers interpret and implement that curriculum. It is now been widely recognised that teaching is a complex process which requires teachers to have knowledge of content, knowledge about pedagogy (how to teach the content), skills and professional attitudes and values (National Institute of Education, 2008). In this respect, an effective teacher training curriculum for HIV and AIDS should include correct and adequate knowledge about HIV and knowledge of the pedagogy of HIV education. Effective teacher training should help teachers '*examine their own attitudes and beliefs regarding sexuality and behaviours towards HIV prevention and gender equality, understand the content they are teaching, learn participatory teaching skills and develop confidence to discuss sensitive topics with young people in their classrooms*' (James-Traore, Finger, Ruland and Savariaud, 2004). Teachers also need to be trained so that they have the awareness and skills to make their classrooms gender responsive (UNESCO, 2004), and to recognise the close relationship between gender socialisation in particular societies and the vulnerability of girls and boys to HIV.

In developing countries, teacher preparation for teaching emerging curricular areas such as HIV and gender are usually carried out through short in-service programmes offered to selected teachers, normally the central department of education. Whatever is learnt through these courses is quickly forgotten and is rarely implemented. Inadequate preparation through short programmes and lack of support and understanding from colleagues, who have not been trained, contribute to this.

Teacher training in these areas needs to be mainstreamed through inclusion in pre-service training. Pre-service courses are of longer duration, normally two years,[2] and accessed by a majority of potential teachers. The trainees are young, at a formative stage of the profession and hence more likely to be open to new ideas and to examining and challenging their existing beliefs. However, as we will report later, the pre-service curriculum is often packed with a lot of content within which content related to HIV and AIDS has a peripheral status.

At a workshop organised by the Commonwealth Secretariat in collaboration with the Association for the Development of Education in Africa (ADEA) in September 2006, two major issues were identified:

- ad hoc teacher training on gender and health which is not integrated into pre- and in-service teacher training systems; and
- ineffective communication of messages to students, parents and communities, especially those dealing with social/religious taboos and discrimination issues.

The workshop recommended a review of teacher development programmes in African countries, so as to incorporate life skills and HIV. We do not have enough knowledge and understanding about how HIV and gender issues are dealt with in pre-service and in-service teacher education programmes in sub-Saharan Africa, nor about how these curricula and practices in Africa can be improved to include and integrate knowledge and strategies for effective HIV, health and gender education.

The review presented in this report was carried out to find out whether and how pre-service teacher education curricula and practices address issues of HIV and gender equality in the three East African countries of Kenya, Tanzania and Uganda.

Chapter 2

Review Methodology

The review is based on three sources:

- Analysis of teacher education policy and curriculum documents from Kenya, Tanzania and Uganda;
- Analysis of teaching/learning materials (where available) used in selected teacher education institutions/colleges in each country; and
- Interviews with a small number of teacher educators and trainee teachers in the selected institutions/colleges in the three countries.

Sample

In each country, we selected six teacher education colleges representing the urban, rural, public and private sectors. The samples from Kenya and Uganda included a large public university as well. This was not possible in Tanzania, where no information was accessible despite consistent efforts by the research team. In each college, group interviews were conducted with six students, while six other students were asked to fill in a questionnaire. In-depth interviews were conducted with four tutors in most colleges. A flexible approach had to be adopted, with group interviews conducted with tutors in some colleges because tutors' schedules did not allow the time required for individual interviews.

Access to curriculum documents and materials was extremely difficult, particularly in Tanzania. These were either not available in colleges or other relevant institutions, or people were reluctant to share them. Nor was it possible to observe teaching practices in any of the colleges, because HIV and gender-related topics were integrated and infused in different subjects and these topics were not being taught during the time of data collection. In some colleges, the trainees and tutors were not sure about when the topics were being taught; in others, the topics had already been taught. In the absence of observation, students and tutors were asked to describe how these topics had been taught in the past.

A consultative workshop was organised from 11 to 13 March 2007 to share the findings of the review with key stakeholders from the three countries, to invite their experiences and perspectives on HIV and gender education, and to provide an opportunity to discuss possibilities of improving teacher preparation for HIV and gender education. Participants of the workshop included the principal and one tutor from each of the colleges in the sample, relevant representatives from the ministries of education in each of the three countries, the review team and a representative from the Commonwealth Secretariat. Overall, the participants confirmed the review findings which highlighted numerous challenges to HIV and AIDS education, in particular resilient cultural beliefs and biases about sexuality and gender, contradictory information about HIV disseminated by different sources (by churches, the media and schools, for example) and gaps between ministry of education policies curricula at primary teachers' colleges (PTCs).

Chapter 3

The Context

The Human Development Index (HDI) provides a measure of a county's development on three dimensions: its people living a long and healthy life, being educated and having a decent standard of living. Countries in sub-Saharan Africa, which include East Africa and the countries within it (Kenya, Tanzania, Uganda and recently added Burundi and Rwanda), rank low on the index. Among the 179 countries for which an HDI is available, Kenya ranks 144, Tanzania 152 and Uganda 156. These countries show high prevalence of HIV and AIDS, although they also show some decline in prevalence since 2001. Nevertheless, the United Nations Programme on HIV and AIDS (UNAIDS) warns that in Uganda, stable HIV trends are occurring alongside an apparent increase in behaviour that favours HIV transmission and a rapidly increasing population, which may increase prevalence levels. National population-based surveys in Tanzania suggest that HIV safe behaviours are declining in some sections of society (UNAIDS, 2008a, p.16).

Table 3.1 Estimated number of people (adults and children) living with HIV

Country	2007 (low and high estimates)	2001 (low and high estimates)
Kenya	1,500,000–2,000,000	1,300,000–1,700,000
Tanzania	1,300,000–1,500,000	1,300,000–1,500,000
Uganda	870,000–100,0000	990,000–1,300,000

Source: Report on the Global AIDS Epidemic, UNAIDS (2008b), p. 214

The rate of HIV and AIDS is substantially higher among young women as compared with young men across all three countries, as seen in table 3.2, below.

Table 3.2 Estimated rate of HIV and AIDS prevalence among young men and women (2007 figures)

Country	% young women (low and high estimates)	% young men (low and high estimates)
Kenya	4.6–8.41	0.8–2.5
Tanzania	0.5–1.3	0.4–0.7
Uganda	2.7–5.2	0.6–1.9

Source: Report on the Global AIDS Epidemic, UNAIDS (2008b), p. 217

Although East African countries have made great gains in removing the gender gap in schools, girls and women in these countries, as well as in sub-Saharan Africa in general, are at a greater risk of acquiring HIV because of socio-economic and cultural attitudes, beliefs and practices (as mentioned above). Studies from many countries in sub-Saharan Africa, including Uganda and Tanzania, suggest that girls and women are economically less independent and develop low self-esteem because of cultural practices. Schools tolerate and promote the power imbalance between girls and boys, which is also reflected in their sexual behaviour. Curricula and teachers promote traditional gender roles and views of male and female sexuality, making girls vulnerable to their fellow male students as well as to male teachers. Even when the school's formal curriculum includes lessons on HIV prevention and awareness of gender issues, teachers' practices and school culture reinforce rather than challenge gendered roles, relationships and practices (Mirambe and Davies, 2001; Vavrus, 2003; Colclough et al., 2003).

Chapter 4

Structure and Scope of School Education in East Africa

Table 4.1 Education in East Africa

Country	Level	Age	Duration
Kenya	Pre-primary	4–6	2
	Primary	6–14	8
	KCSE	14–18	4
	Tertiary	18+	4
Tanzania	Pre-primary	4–6	2
	Primary	7–13	7
	CSE	14–17	4
	CASE	18–20	2
	Tertiary	20+	3
Uganda	Pre-primary	3–5	3
	Primary	6–12	7
	UCE	13–16	4
	UACE	17–18	2
	Tertiary	19+	3

KCSE: Kenya Certificate of Secondary Education
CSE: Certificate of Secondary Education
CASE: Certificate of Advanced Secondary Education
UCE: Uganda Certificate of Education
UACE: Uganda Advanced Certificate of Education

Kenya

Kenya attained independence in 1963 from the British government. The new government undertook the provision of education and training as key to overall national development. To address the challenges facing the education sector, a commission of education chaired by Professor Simon Ominde was formed to reform the education system inherited from the colonial government to meet the country's needs (ROK, 1964). Since then, the challenges facing the education sector have been addressed through commissions, committees and taskforces. This commission proposed an education system that would foster national unity and the creation of sufficient human capital for national development. Kenya's current education system was put in place in 1981, as a result of a Presidential Working Party Report on the second university in Kenya (ROK, 1981), which led to the establishment of the 8.4.4 system of education. The system includes three years early childhood development education (ECDE), two years pre-primary, eight years primary and four years secondary/technical education (see table 4.1).

Kenya's Ministry of Education, Science and Technology (MOEST) is charged with developing education policy documents. Current education policy is based on the recommendations of the National Conference on Education and Training, which was held in November 2003. The theme of the conference, Meeting the Challenges of Education and Training in Kenya in the 21st Century, reflects the government's continued pursuit of relevant education. The conference was held against a backdrop of challenges facing the education sector, which were listed as access, equity, quality and relevance.

The overall policy goal of the Kenyan government is to achieve Education For All (EFA). The priority is to ensure equitable access and improvements in quality and efficiency at all levels of education. The ultimate goal is to develop an all inclusive and quality education that is accessible and relevant to all Kenyans. This is guided by the understanding that good education can contribute significantly to economic growth, improved employment prospects and income generating opportunities (MOEST, 2004).

Tanzania

The school system in Tanzania comprises two years pre-primary, seven years primary education, four years secondary education (leading to the Certificate of Secondary Education Examination [CSEE]) and an additional two years of advanced secondary education (leading to the Certificate of

Advanced Secondary Education Examination [CASEE]). Pre-primary education is not compulsory and is offered mainly by private schools. At primary school, children are required to study Kiswahili, English, mathematics, social studies, science, life skills and religious instruction as compulsory subjects. At the secondary level, students must take six compulsory subjects and at least one subject from their chosen stream. They can choose from agriculture, commerce, arts and science streams.

Students may undertake vocational and professional training after completing primary education. Those who complete upper secondary (advanced level or 'A-levels') can join either tertiary or higher education and vocational training institutions or enter the job market. There are more than 140 tertiary training institutions in Tanzania, and some 33 of these are higher education institutions, categorised into universities (eight public and 12 private) and university colleges (four public and nine private).

The government, through its Ministry of Education and Vocational Training (MEVT), is the main provider of school education. However, there is a growing number of private and non-governmental organisation (NGO)-managed schools.

There has been a substantial increase in primary school enrolment since the Tanzanian government made primary education compulsory and free: some 2.2 million additional learners enrolled between 2001 and 2004. In 2006, the gross and net enrolment ratios (GER,[3] NER) for primary schools were 117.7 per cent and 96.1 per cent respectively. Eighty-seven per cent of children continue in school to grade 5 and 74 per cent complete grade 7 (2006). Enrolment at secondary level is low, but has shown improvement and has doubled since 2000. In 2006, the secondary school GER was 14.8 per cent and the NER was 13.0 per cent.

The official recommendation for the teacher-pupil ratio in Tanzania's schools is 1:45. However, the actual average teacher-student ratio in primary schools is 1:52 and can go as high as 1:90 in some districts.

Uganda

Pre-primary education is mainly managed by private agencies and individuals. Most nursery schools and kindergartens are concentrated in urban areas, where a large percentage of parents can afford to pay and appreciate the value of such education. Primary education terminates at grade 7 with the Primary Leaving Examination Certificate. The focus of the examination is English, mathematics, science and social studies.

Secondary education comprises four years of lower secondary (ordinary level) leading to the Uganda Certificate of Education and two years of upper secondary (advanced level) leading to the Uganda Advanced Certificate of Education. Technical schools are alternatives to secondary education. Both primary and secondary school leavers study technical education for three years, with the curriculum including various crafts and vocational skills. Some technical and commercial institutes are privately owned. However, opportunities in vocational education are restricted due to the high cost of establishing and maintaining basic facilities (Ministry of Education and Sports [MOES], 2006a).

In Uganda, the terms 'tertiary' and 'higher education' are used synonymously to refer to post-secondary education offered in universities, polytechnics, institutes, colleges and other institutes affiliated to these. There are five public and more than 25 licensed private universities, which award various degrees (National Council for Higher Education [NCHE], 2006). The government sponsors about 4,000 students each year for different courses in public universities. There is also significant investment by the private sector (including NGOs) in higher education (MOES, 2006a). More students are enrolled in private universities than in public universities.

The Ministry of Education and Sports (MOES) provides, supports, guides, co-ordinates, regulates and promotes quality education and sports to all persons in Uganda for national integration, individual and national development. Although the government endeavours to provide public schooling for all Ugandans, government-aided schools are insufficient in number and so public education is offered through private schools affiliated to religious organisations and those owned by educational entrepreneurs. The MOES regulates education in private schools.

Compared to pre-primary (4 per cent) and secondary education (19 per cent), primary school enrolment is high (119 per cent) (MOES, 2006b). Primary education in Uganda has thrived since the introduction of universal primary education (UPE) in 1997. In 2005, over 7.7 million children of primary school-going age attended school (MOES, 2006b). However, only 49 per cent of children who begin school complete five years of schooling and only 25 per cent complete the last grade of school. The teacher-student ratio is high in primary schools, averaging 1:52 – although there are some classrooms with up to 250 children.

Chapter 5

Structure and Scope of Pre-service Teacher Education in East Africa

An appropriate level of pre-service training is normally required for appointment as a school teacher in Kenya, Tanzania and Uganda, and this is mostly delivered by government-funded teacher training colleges (TTCs) and universities. Privately funded institutions are relatively few and often affiliated with religious organisations. Of the three countries, Tanzania has the highest number of teacher training colleges and also the highest number of privately owned institutions (46 public and 13 private). Uganda has 49 colleges, only two of which are privately owned, and Kenya has 21 public and nine private teacher education colleges.

In each country, a certificate in teaching is normally required to teach at primary level, while a diploma is required to teach at secondary level and a degree is preferred to teach upper secondary (or A-level). The entry-level requirement for the certificate course is a minimum of four years secondary education (O-levels). In Uganda and Tanzania, entry to diploma programmes requires six years of secondary education (A-levels), while in Kenya, where secondary school comprises four rather than six years, a minimum of C+ at secondary school examination is required. Curricula for the certificate and diploma courses are prepared centrally: by the Kenya Institute of Education (KIE) in Kenya, by the Tanzania Institute of Education (TIE) in Tanzania and by MOES/Kyambogo University in Uganda.

A Bachelor of Education (BEd) degree is offered by most universities in the three countries. In recent years, specialised degrees in education have become possible, such as a BEd in early childhood and development, BEd in library studies and a BEd in educational communication and technology. Uganda is the only country among the three that offers a degree in technical teacher education and that has a department of teacher education and development studies at a public university.

Table 5.1 Teacher training and certification in Kenya, Uganda and Tanzania

	Kenya	Uganda	Tanzania
Certificate programmes	Primary teacher certificate (2 yrs) Offered by TTC[4]	Grade 3 primary teacher certificate (2 yrs) Offered by TTC	Certificate in teaching (2 yrs) Offered by TTC
Diploma programmes	Diploma in education (2 yrs) Postgraduate diploma in education (1 yr) Offered by universities	Diploma in education (2 yrs) Offered by NTC[5] Postgraduate diploma in education (1 yr) Offered by universities	Diploma in teaching (2 yrs) Postgraduate diploma in education (1 yr) Offered by TTC
Degree programmes	Bachelor of Education (4 yrs) Offered by universities	Bachelor of Education (3 yrs) Offered by universities	Bachelor of Education (3 yrs) Offered by universities

Chapter 6

The Policy Context for HIV and Gender Education

East African countries declared HIV and AIDS a national disaster during the 1990s; for Uganda this declaration was as early as 1992, while in Kenya and Tanzania it took place as late as 1999. These declarations were followed by a number of policies, plans and institutional structures to lead and co-ordinate prevention and care.

The initial response to the epidemic was primarily a medical one. However, during the 1990s the realisation that HIV is a multi-sector issue became evident in policies and plans. In these it was recognised not only that the education sector had been severely affected by HIV, but also that education has the strongest potential to improve prevention and care. Policies and plans recommend that HIV education should be mainstreamed by integrating it into the school curricula at both primary and secondary levels. They also refer to the need for HIV and AIDS education for teachers. Of the three countries under review, Kenya's policy is most explicit on integrating such education into its teacher training curricula.

Kenya

Kenya launched an education sector policy on HIV in 2004, emphasising the responsibility of all learning institutions to address HIV through education by developing skills and values and changing attitudes to promote positive behaviour. It recommends mainstreaming HIV education in school curricula and co-curricular activities, and preparing teachers 'to respond to HIV and AIDS within their own lives and as professionals to build positive attitudes and skills for HIV and AIDS prevention and control among their learners' (MOEST, 2005).

Kenya's national gender and development policy was formulated by the

Ministry of Gender, Sports, Culture and Social Services (MGSC&SS) in 2000, with the purpose of mainstreaming gender into development projects as well as reviewing previous strategies which were based on traditional assumptions of the roles and responsibilities of women and men (MGSC& SS, 2000, p. 6). The policy recognises current gender disparities in Kenya, and recommends measures to eliminate gender disparities in access, retention, transition and performance in education for both boys and girls. In 2001, a Technical Sub-Committee on Gender and HIV and AIDS Task Force recommended gender mainstreaming in all initiatives to respond to HIV.

Tanzania

Tanzania developed a national policy on HIV in 2001. This policy recommends that non-examinable information on HIV, reproductive and sexual health should be included in primary and secondary school curricula. A national multi-sectoral framework developed in 2003 expects the education sector to require primary and secondary schools to provide '*education and opportunities for young people to develop and maintain orientations, values, attitudes and activities which safeguard their sexual and reproductive health*'. The framework also proposes integration of sexual health for young people into the curricula for teacher training.

Uganda

In Uganda, the national overarching policy on HIV and the national strategic plan framework urge the development of sector-specific policies. The education sector policy and guidelines, drafted in 2004, set out some principals, goals and strategies for prevention, treatment and care and support. The principles include mainstreaming HIV into every policy, procedure and programme in the education sector and providing universal access to education, information and communication about the issue to reduce the vulnerability of learners and education sector personnel. The policy recommends mainstreaming and integrating life skills education and HIV into the curricula of all learning institutions and building capacity for providing basic AIDS education.

Each of the three countries have also formulated national gender policies that aim to guide the initiatives to redress gender imbalance, ensure equal access to resources and to promote recognition of women's role in development. Various policies, including the education policy in each country, express a commitment to taking initiatives to increase and improve girls' and women's participation in education.

Chapter 7
Teacher Education Curriculum

In response to the policies discussed above, HIV and AIDS education has been infused and integrated into the teacher education curricula in each of the three countries reviewed. This integration is more explicit in Kenya and Tanzania, where the curricula have recently been revised (in 2004 and 2007 respectively) than in Uganda, where the current curricula (revised in 1994) does not explicitly include HIV education in its objectives or content. Uganda's revised primary teacher training curriculum will become available in 2009. The following sections describe and discuss integration and infusion of HIV education and gender education into the curricula of each country and identify similarities and differences between them.

Kenya

In Kenya, the primary teacher education curriculum has six main objectives. While none of the six address HIV or gender directly, one relates to health education: to '*develop in the teacher awareness and appreciation for good health and environmental conservation*'. Gender education is not addressed at all in the curricular objectives, nor is it integrated in any of the subject syllabi. However, one of the country's eight National Goals for Education relates to gender education indirectly. This goal states that '*Education in Kenya should promote social equity and responsibility. It should give all children varied and challenging opportunities for collective activities and corporate social service irrespective of gender, ability or geographical environment*' (MOEST, 2004).

Kenya's primary teacher education (PTE) curriculum is spread over two years. In the first year trainees are required to study ten compulsory subjects (see table 7.1, below). The introductory comments and the general objectives identified for each of the ten courses make reference to HIV and include the objective of integrating and infusing HIV, gender and other cross-cutting issues. However, these are not translated into the recommended content and no instruction is given on how to infuse these when teaching other topics. For example, in physical education, '*Trainees are expected to be able to express a variety of themes on contemporary issues such as gender issues and HIV and AIDS through movement*'. In the first instance, this is a very vague objective, and in the second, it is not included in the specific objectives and content of the syllabus. Teaching methodology and teaching resources are recommended for each subject, but they are merely listed. The list includes participatory approaches such as story telling, play activities, role play, miming, dramatisation, lectures, educational visits, case studies, questions and answers, brain storming and debate (MOEST, 2004). However, the syllabus does not explicitly link these methods with any particular content. There is obviously an expectation that tutors will be able to use appropriate and relevant teaching methodology. That this is an unrealistic expectation becomes evident as we examine practice in the colleges.

Table 7.1 Organisation of the primary teacher education (PTE) syllabus in Kenya

Session	Subjects offered
Year one	1. Mathematics, including aspects of business studies 2. English, including aspects of library science, native language and drama 3. Kiswahili, including aspects of library science, native language and drama 4. Science, integrated with home science and agriculture 5. Religious education (Christian and Islamic religious education [CRE/IRE]) 6. Social studies, including some aspects of business studies 7. Education, including special needs educations 8. Creative arts (integrated music, art and craft, and drama) 9. Physical education 10. Information and communication technology (ICT) 11. One session of teaching practice
	Five core subjects
Year two	1. English 2. Kiswahili 3. Education 4. Physical Education 5. ICT

Table 7.1 (continued)

OPTION A	OPTION B
• Science • Home science • Agriculture • Mathematics	• Music • Art and craft • Social studies • Religious education
Two sessions of teaching practice	

In the second year, trainees must study five core and compulsory subjects and four elective subjects to specialise in either science (option A) or humanities (option B), with two teaching practice sessions in their chosen option. HIV and gender appear in the general goals and objectives of the five compulsory subjects, but are not carried through into the content or methodology in any significant way. The main carrier subjects for HIV are science and home economics within option A and social studies and religious education within option B (see table 7.2 below).

The syllabi for science and home science are concerned with providing scientific factual knowledge about transmission, prevention and care. The science syllabus aims to enable students to learn to:

> *'Define HIV and AIDS, describe modes of transmission, stages of development, testing and counselling for HIV and AIDS, identifying the myths and misconceptions about HIV and AIDS, state ways of demystifying myths and misconceptions about HIV and AIDS, explain ways of caring for those affected and infected by HIV and AIDS, list down different ways of controlling HIV and AIDS, state the impact of HIV and AIDS on the individual, the family and the nation, know about the proper nutrition for special groups such as people living with HIV and AIDS'* (MOEST, 2004, vol. 2, p. 36–7, 50).

The home science syllabus focuses on home-based care for the sick. Students are expected to learn to:

> *'Define home-based care, state reasons for caring for the sick at home, explain how to care for the sick at home, observe/measure when taking care of the sick at home (to include HIV and AIDS), importance of voluntary counselling and testing (VCT) in HIV and AIDS, safety measures to be observed by traditional birth attendants (TBAs) during delivery in relation to HIV and*

Table 7.2 Carrier subjects and integrated HIV content in the 2004 primary teacher education (PTE) syllabus in Kenya

Subject/topic	Objectives	Content	Proposed method/resources
Subject: Science Topic: **Health education, food & nutrition** Vol. 2, pp. 29–117	**At the end of this topic the learner should be able to:** • Define HIV and AIDS; describe modes of transmission, stages of development, testing and counselling for HIV and AIDS • Identify the myths and misconceptions about HIV; state ways of demystifying these myths and misconceptions • Explain ways of caring for those affected and infected by HIV and AIDS • List different ways of controlling HIV • State the impact of HIV on the individual, the family and the nation (pp. 36–38) • Describe the nutrition for different special groups	Definition of HIV and AIDS; modes of transmission, stages of development, counselling and testing; myths and misconceptions, care and support for those infected and affected; control of HIV; impact of HIV on the individual, family and the nation (Vol. 2, pp. 36–37) Food & nutrition and HIV: Vol. 2, p. 50 First aid and HIV: Vol. 2, p. 93 Health care: VCT (Vol. 2, p. 108) Confinement: TBAs (Vol. 2, p. 110) Home-based care: Vol. 2, p. 94 Nutrition for special groups: pregnant and lactating mothers, infants, people living with HIV and AIDS	**Teaching and learning resources** suggested include real objects, posters, charts, pictures/photographs, magazines, resource persons, newspapers, audio tapes, films, slides, tools, the environment, condoms, immunisation cards and ICT (Vol. 2, pp. 64–65) Suggested **teaching methods** for science: observation, demonstration, discussion, question and answer, drawing, practicals, visits, science walks, experimentation and a science kit (Vol. 2 p. 65) Suggested assessment methods: observation, oral questioning, written tests and project work

Table 7.2 (continued)

Subject/topic	Objectives	Content	Proposed method/resources
Mathematics Vol. 2, pp. 1–28	**At the end of the course the learner should be able to:** • Relate mathematical concepts to real life situations, including emerging issues (Vol. 2, p. 2)	No specific content mentioned	Emerging issues such as HIV, gender, integrity and human rights will be addressed in the process of problem solving (Vol. 1, p. 1)
Creative arts Vol. 1, pp. 140–207	**At the end of the course the learner should be able to:** • Infuse emerging issues related to child labour, drug abuse, HIV, integrity, human rights, environment and gender (Vol. 1, p. 141) **Vol. 1, p. 141: Creative – introduction** ... 'the content has also been carefully selected to infuse emerging issues related to child labour, drug abuse, HIV and AIDS, integrity, human rights, the environment and gender' ...	**Vol. 1, p. 179: Practical – specific objectives** Topical songs on: Child labour, HIV, drug abuse, integrity, environmental issues, human rights, gender and corruption	Lyrics of songs on various issues such as: HIV, integrity, corruption, child rights, drug abuse, environmental issues, human rights (Vol. 1, p. 180)

Table 7.2 (continued)

Subject/topic	Objectives	Content	Proposed method/resources
Information and communication technology Vol.1, pp. 208–235	Teachers today live in a society where there is immense pressure to address emerging issues. The introduction of the Internet, therefore, will be particularly useful as a source of information for teachers in addressing issues such as: HIV, drug abuse, the environment, gender issues and child labour (Vol. 1, p. 209)	The Internet as a source of information on emerging issues such as: HIV, drug abuse, gender issues and child labour (Vol. 1, p. 209)	A list of teaching and learning experiences are given at the end of the content ... none is given specifically to address issues related to HIV
Physical education Vol. 1, pp. 79–108	**At the end of this topic the learner should be able to:** • Express themselves on a variety of themes such as drug abuse, gender issues, HIV and integrity	Movement (Vol. 1, p. 81)	
Social studies Vol. 1, pp. 108–139	**At the end of this topic the learner should be able to:** • Explain the effects of HIV on population growth in Kenya (Vol. 1, p. 119)	Content includes the effects of HIV on population growth in Kenya (Vol. 1, p. 120); care and support of family members with special needs such as HIV, disabilities, drug and substance abuse (Vol. 1, p. 121)	List of teaching and learning experiences are given at the end of the content

Table 7.2 (continued)

Subject/topic	Objectives	Content	Proposed method/resources
Social studies (continued)	**Vol. 1, p. 110: Social studies – introduction** ... 'the emerging issues relating to HIV and AIDS, drug and substance abuse, integrity, gender, legal aspects, human have been addressed through movement'. **General objectives:** No mention of HIV, though it is implied in objective number 9 under social justice and number 12: contemporary issues	**Vol. 1, p. 119: Peoples and population – specific objectives** 'explain the effects of HIV and AIDS on population growth in Kenya' **Vol. 1, p. 120: Content** 'Effects of HIV and AIDS on population growth in Kenya' **Vol. 1, p. 120: Social organisations, institutions and cultural activities – specific objectives** Care and support of family members with special needs: • HIV and AIDS • Disabilities • Drug and substance abuse	
Education Vol. 2, pp. 118–147	**Introduction:** Emerging issues such as HIV, integrity and drug and substance abuse have also been integrated and infused. This is to enable learners to be responsive to critical issues affecting society (p. 119) **At the end of the course, the learner should be able to:**	Content includes: • Children with special needs, intervention measures for children with special needs • Counselling issues in primary schools and referrals (behavioural problems, developmental problems, relationships, emotional/	**Teaching:** Role play (p. 146) Observation, lectures, research, educational visits, demonstrations, discussions, question and answer, group work, assignments (p. 147) **Resources:** reference books, resource persons, pictures, charts, realia, audio-visual aids, case studies

Table 7.2 (continued)

Subject/topic	Objectives	Content	Proposed method/resources
Education (continued)	• **General objectives:** Develop in the child appreciation for good health and environmental care, identify and provide support for children with psychosocial difficulties, acquire basic theoretical and practical knowledge about sociological issues that affect education (p. 120) • **Specific objectives:** Identify and discuss counselling issues in primary schools • **Sociology of education:** specific objectives: explain the socio-economic problems in education (p. 140)	psychological problems, HIV, special needs, academic achievement (p. 138) • Sociology of education: socio-economic problems in education in relation to: HIV, children living in difficult circumstances, drug and substance abuse, social stratification, corruption (p. 140)	
Christian religious education Vol. 2, pp. 148–174	**At the end of the course, the learner should be able to:** • **Knowledge:** identify contemporary issues that affect the teacher trainee's life and those of the pupils • **Skills:** use life skills to cope with challenges of a rapidly changing society (p. 151), explain the skills required for healthy living, desire to develop life skills (p. 160)	Content includes: • Effects of irresponsible sexual behaviour (p. 171), HIV and sexually transmitted diseases (Vol. 2, p. 170) • **Life skills:** knowing and living with oneself (self awareness, self esteem, coping with emotions, coping with challenges, p. 160), knowing and living with others	Story telling, role play, visits, discussions, projects, dramatisation and discovery. Also question and answer, miming, song, dance, drawing, modelling, demonstrations, recitation, memorisation (p. 164) **Resource:** *The Bible*

Table 7.2 (continued)

Subject/topic	Objectives	Content	Proposed method/resources
Christian religious education (continued)	• **Contemporary Christian living:** explain the meaning of human sexuality, explain the traditional African view on human sexuality, explain Christian teaching on human sexuality, identify forms and causes of irresponsible sexual behaviour, discuss Christian responsibility to those affected by irresponsible sexual behaviour, describe Christian teaching on marriage and family, discuss the traditional African view on marriage and family, state the problems affecting the family today, discuss the responsibility of parents towards their children, appreciate Christian teaching on responsible sexual behaviour, discuss how leisure is misused in society (p. 170)	(assertiveness, empathy/sharing, negotiation/tolerance, effective communication, conflict resolution, p. 161), making effective decisions (critical thinking, creative thinking, decision-making, p. 161) • **Contemporary Christian living:** meaning of human sexuality, the traditional African view on human sexuality, Christian teaching on human sexuality (Genesis 1: 22–27, Psalms 139: 13–15), irresponsible sexual behaviour (Romans 1: 22–27), effects of irresponsible sexual behaviour: HIV and sexually transmitted diseases, early pregnancies, early marriage, school drop-outs, guilt, stress (1 Corinthians: 6: 12–20), Christian responsibility to those affected by irresponsible sexual behaviour (p. 171), misuse of leisure: drug and substance abuse, sexual immorality, pornography (p. 172)	

Table 7.2 (continued)

Subject/topic	Objectives	Content	Proposed method/resources
Islamic religious education Vol. 2, pp. 175–195	**At the end of this topic the learner should be able to:** • Respond and adapt to contemporary issues facing society from an Islamic perspective (p. 177) • Integrate and infuse contemporary issues	Content includes: • **Moral values:** Islamic teaching on chastity, sexual behaviour, HIV (p. 179) • Drug and substance abuse, environmental issues, etc. (Vol. 2, p. 189) • *Muamalat* (relationships), care and services for the sick (care for people living with AIDS [PLWA]) (Vol. 2, p. 193)	**Teaching/learning experiences:** Discussion, explanation, narration, memorisation, role play, question and answer, deduction, dramatisation, project work, brainstorming, visits, case studies, debates, demonstrations (p. 195) **Resources:** Holy *Qur'an*, resource persons, collection of *Hadith*, audio-visual aids, print media models, real objects
Home science Vol. 2, pp. 90–117	**At the end of the topic, the learner should be able to:** • **First Aid:** observe safety measures when giving first aid (p. 93), observe safety measures to include HIV when taking care of the sick at home (p. 94) • **Mother and child health care:** explain preparation for parenthood, explain the importance of voluntary counselling and testing (VCT) when preparing for parenthood	Content includes: • **First Aid:** safety measures when giving First Aid to include HIV (p. 93) • **Home-based care:** definition, reasons for caring for the sick at home (giving medicine, nutrition, feeding, bathing, clothing and bedding, utensils, cleaning the room, equipment, and materials used by the patient), safety measures to observe when caring for the sick at home	**Cleaning equipment and materials:** water heater, basins, buckets, dustpan, brooms, brushes (cloths, scrubbing, shoe brush, cobweb brush) **Safety equipment:** first aid kit **Suggested teaching/learning experiences:** discussion, visits, demonstrations, question and answer, observation, project work, practicals, role play (p. 117)

Table 7.2 (continued)

Subject/topic	Objectives	Content	Proposed method/resources
Home science (continued)		• **Mother and child health care:** preparation for parenthood (physical, psychological, social, economic), importance of VCT in HIV and AIDS, needs of an expectant mother (diet, rest, clothing and shoes, emotional support), services offered at antenatal clinic, postnatal care (importance, services offered at postnatal clinic, health and growth monitoring chart) **p. 110: Confinement – content** Safety measures to be observed by traditional birth assistants (TBAs) during delivery in relation to HIV	

> *AIDS. Nutrition for special groups: pregnant and lactating mothers … people living with HIV and AIDS'.*

Within option B, the syllabi for social and religious education include objectives and content related to the psycho-social aspects of HIV. The specific HIV-related objectives and content of the social studies syllabus focus on '*the effects of HIV and AIDS on population growth and the care and support of family members with special needs, including the needs of those with HIV and AIDS*'. The objectives of the Islamic and Christian religious education syllabi include the acquisition of knowledge of contemporary issues, including HIV and AIDS, which affect life and relationships and the skills required to cope with these issues. Content such life skills and moral and religious values for responsible sexual behaviour and healthy living, and responsibilities for the care and service of the sick are included.

The HIV-related content in the syllabi of the carrier subjects is oriented towards giving basic knowledge and awareness to future teachers. The application of this knowledge in their personal lives is not explicit, except perhaps in religious education and in the core course on education. In this later course, guidance and counselling and sociology of education appear as topics. Within these topics, trainees are expected to discuss counselling issues in primary schools in relation to HIV, and to study HIV as one of several socio-economic problems in education.

The integration of different aspects of HIV education in the specialised/elective subjects (rather in most core subjects) means that those who take the science option will acquire factual knowledge about transmission, prevention and care, while those who opt for humanities will develop understanding of the social effects of HIV and moral and religious responsibilities that affect sexual behaviour. Having elective subjects as the main carriers reduces the impact of integration. Future teachers will not have the holistic knowledge, skills and attitudes required to change personal behaviour or to influence the behaviour of young people in schools, as envisaged by Kenya's education sector policy on HIV, 2004.

Universities in Kenya follow general education policies and guidelines prescribed by the central government, but devise their own programme of studies. We could not obtain information from every university in Kenya; however, we did approach one of the largest public universities, located in Nairobi. At this university, HIV education is a stand alone, compulsory and examinable course for all students in pre-service teacher education programmes. The grade obtained in this course counts towards the overall grade obtained in the BEd degree. Faculty members have prepared the course outline and materials (including a textbook), and the content includes basic scientific information on adolescent development, fertility, sexually transmitted diseases (STDs), HIV – its nature, modes of transmission and management. The course also includes the social and personal implications of HIV, such as its impact on families and organisations, and social and cultural beliefs and practices which contribute to the spread. Unlike the syllabi in the certificate programme described earlier, which do not deal with how to teach HIV in school, the university curriculum does include topics on approaches to HIV education, such as the participatory mode and peer education.

Since the launch of the policy, MOEST has worked with other non-governmental organisations like the Centre for British Teachers (CfBT) to implement school-based HIV education and behaviour-change interventions through the Primary School Action for Better Health (PSABH). MOEST and CfBT use a cascade model, in which they train a principal (or deputy) and two tutors. The trained tutors then train their colleagues and provide HIV and AIDS education in the classrooms and organise co-curricular activities in their institutions using materials and resources provided by CfBT. In two of the colleges visited, the principal and two tutors had gone through the programme.

Tanzania

As mentioned earlier in this report, three types of pre-service programmes provide pre-service teacher education in Tanzania: certificate, diploma and degree programmes. The certificate and diploma programmes prepare most school teachers in the country (see table 7.3, below) and hence we review the syllabi for these two courses below.

Table 7.3 Number of teachers trained through different teacher education programmes in Tanzania

	Public schools			Private schools			Total		
	Male	Female	Total	M	F	T	M	F	T
BSc (Ed)	575	170	745	524	156	680	1,099	326	1,425
BSc (Gen)	234	77	311	257	62	319	491	139	630
BA (Ed)	717	213	930	973	254	1,227	1,690	467	2,157
BA (Gen)	231	67	298	467	60	527	698	127	825
Dip. Science	4,158	1,726	5,884	1,831	418	2,249	5,989	2,144	8,133
Dip. Arts	4,873	2,931	7,804	2,256	718	2,974	7,129	3,649	10,778
Grade A	409	330	739	188	70	258	597	400	997
Others	546	96	642	1,931	333	2,264	2,477	429	2,906
Total	12,339	5,885	18,224	9,072	2,181	11,253	21,411	8,066	29,477

From: Lewin (2003)

The certificate in teaching curriculum lists seven objectives, only one of which addresses HIV and gender directly, along with other issues. This objective states that the certificate course will '*enable pre-service teachers to enhance their understanding of national and international issues, particularly HIV and AIDS education, gender, children's rights and conservation of the environment*'.

Trainees must study 11 compulsory subjects, with topics relating to HIV and gender integrated in five of these (see table 7.4, below). So although HIV education does not appear as a specific topic or as a focused objective, it is infused within other topics such as adolescence and youth problems, gender and cross-cutting issues. For example, the syllabus for the subject of guidance and counselling recommends that trainees discuss youth problems such as being affected by HIV. The civics syllabus recommends class discussion on the effects of widow inheritance on the spread of HIV. Widow inheritance is a common practice in some parts of Africa, whereby a widowed woman is taken over by a brother or cousin of her dead husband.

Table 7.4 Analysis of the certificate course in teacher education

Subject	Topic	Objectives	Proposed methods	Resources
Psychology, guidance and counselling	• Child growth and development • Types of child growth • Youth and adolescence	• Trainee should be able to elaborate how gender equality contributes to child development • Trainee should be able to define and describe adolescent problems and ways of building good behaviour	• In groups, trainees discuss effects of gender bias on children's upbringing • Trainees discuss problems that adolescents face, including using drugs, becoming affected by HIV, living responsibly, imitating and copying	• Immunisation card • Child development programme • Books showing nutritional charts • Books on parts of the body
Social studies, teaching and learning methods	• Division of labour in the family • Roles and responsibilities in the family • Norms and behaviour of Tanzanians	• To explain the concept of division of labour • To identify appropriate divisions of labour • To identify the possibility of gender inequality • Identify cultural practices which perpetuate gender inequality	• Tutors use a division of labour chart to guide learners to identify division of labour for each family member • Use of role play • Use of brainstorming • Group discussions	• Pictures of family members at work • Division of labour chart • Chart on roles and responsibilities • TV • Charts
Civics	• Gender issues	• To explain the meaning of gender and gender equality • To explain violations of gender equality in Tanzanian culture • To be aware of discrimination against women and girls	• Discussion through question and answer • Discussion on violations of gender equality by the practice of gender[6] mutilation and widow inheritance	• Newspapers with news on gender • Video on HIV and AIDS

Table 7.4 (continued)

Subject	Topic	Objectives	Proposed methods	Resources
Civics (continued)		• Explain how gender inequality hinders economic growth • State strategies for bringing about gender equality • To explain the importance of NGOs and civil society in strengthening gender equality • Elaborate on the importance of both men and women in promoting and strengthening gender equality	• Discussion of the effect of widow inheritance on the spread of HIV and oppression of women • Group discussions to suggest strategies for promoting gender equality • Discussions on the importance of men and women	
Science	• Disease	• To be able to explain the spread of disease by air, water and contact • Explain how to protect from various diseases	• Brainstorming to identify infectious diseases such as HIV, malaria etc. • Discuss how to protect oneself	• Use items from the environment
Mathematics				
Kiswahili	• Riddles • Stories	• Identify riddles with gender bias • Identify gender bias in stories		

Table 7.4 (continued)

Subject	Topic	Objectives	Proposed methods	Resources
Curriculum and teaching				
Foundations of education	• Explain the importance of topics on cross-cutting issues	• Question and answer to explain concept of cross-cutting issues • Trainees discuss cross-cutting issues such as HIV and gender to explain their importance		
Teaching learning methods				
Early childhood care and development				
Research measurement and evaluation				

Various resources such as books, charts and videos are recommended for tutors to use in the training. However, no particular books or resource materials are prescribed and, as our discussion of practice suggests (below), not all colleges have similar quantities or quality of resources and other learning materials. Discussion and brainstorming among trainees are recommended as the main learning methods so as to encourage participation.

Where it appears as a topic, civics is the primary carrier subject for gender. Teacher trainees are expected to become aware of violations of gender equality in Tanzanian culture and discrimination against women and girls. They are also expected to be able to state strategies for bringing about gender equality, and to explain the importance of NGOs, civil societies and men and women in bringing gender equality. The syllabi for social studies and psychology and for guidance and counselling (which is one subject) also include gender-related objectives and content. In social studies, for example, students are expected to be able to identify gender inequality as part of studying family roles, responsibilities and norms. In psychology, guidance and counselling trainees are expected to elaborate how gender equality contributes to child development as an outcome of studying child growth and types of child growth. The syllabi for Kiswahili and foundations of education suggest that teachers infuse gender awareness while teaching other topics – for example, identify riddles with gender bias.

These gender-related objectives across the subjects seem to focus on awareness of an existing situation of gender inequality, so that trainee teachers can identify, explain or elaborate gender inequality in the family and in cultural practices. However, they do not expect trainees to examine their own beliefs, attitudes or experiences, or to learn to become more gender sensitive as teachers in their own classrooms. The syllabus proposes discussion as the primary method of teaching, and suggests a variety of resources to be made available in the colleges. Yet materials on gender were largely absent.

In terms of the diploma in teaching, Tanzania's two-year Diploma in Secondary Education comprises both compulsory and specialisation subjects. All students must take the following compulsory subjects: foundations of education; curriculum and teaching; development studies, educational psychology, guidance and counselling; educational research and management; and communication skills. Students must also specialise in one of the following subjects: biology, physics, chemistry, mathematics, civics, geography, history, Kiswahili, English, information and computer studies or French. Each of these specialisation subjects has an academic (focusing on subject matter) and a pedagogy syllabus. For each syllabus, the Tanzania Institute of Education (TIE) has developed a module as a resource for students. In the discussion below, we refer to these modules along with the syllabus document. Information obtained from the sample colleges, however, suggested that the modules were not available in all colleges.

Gender and HIV appear as topics primarily in one of the compulsory subjects (development studies) and are included rather minimally in the syllabus for foundations of education (see table 7.5, below). The syllabus for the latter recommends that gender and HIV should be discussed as two of the nine factors influencing education. However, the module for this subject does not include any reference to gender or HIV, nor does it suggest any activities to discuss the influence of these two factors on education in Tanzania.

The development studies syllabus includes HIV and gender as specific topics within the broader theme of 'theories and aspects of development'. Four hours are allocated to the teaching of HIV, so as to enable trainees to determine the extent of the disease in Tanzania, assess the effectiveness of prevention strategies and point out how to avoid risk behaviour. The module on this subject provides some basic information on the prevalence of HIV and AIDS in the world and in Tanzania. It also lists the most vulnerable groups and prevention strategies: abstinence, self-control, counselling, testing, prevention of mother-child transmission and school-based prevention at primary and secondary level. No further explanations are given on this list. The module recommends that trainees use the information provided in the module to educate their students and provide guidance and counselling to the infected and affected members of the community, but does not give any input on how to do this or the pedagogy of HIV education.

The module also includes three so-called 'activities', although they primarily require trainees to answer questions such as 'What is the HIV/AIDS epidemic?' and 'How is it transmitted?' Another 'activity' requires trainees to discuss which risk behaviours lead to HIV infection, and to assess which strategies are effective in alleviating HIV-related problems in their locality. No information is given in the module to help answer these questions, suggesting that the student teachers and the tutors themselves are

Table 7.5 Analysis of the diploma course in teacher education

Course title, objectives and competencies	Topic and time allocated	Topic-specific objectives	Teaching and learning strategies	Teaching and learning resources
Curriculum and teaching: • Integrate cross-cutting issues into the teaching and learning process				
Foundations of education: • Acquire knowledge and develop understanding of educational equality and equity in education • Identify and integrate cross-cutting issues in area of specialisation	Sociological factors influencing education in Tanzania: 3 hours	• Identify and analyse sociological factors that influence education in Tanzania • Explain basic ideas of distinguished sociologists • Apply sociological ideas	• Small group discussions on the factors; HIV and gender included among nine factors listed	• Newspaper cuttings, encyclopaedia of sociology and education, test materials on sociological factors
Educational research and management				

Table 7.5 (continued)

Course title, objectives and competencies	Topic and time allocated	Topic-specific objectives	Teaching and learning strategies	Teaching and learning resources
Development studies: • Identify, evaluate and propose solutions for socio-economic problems • Develop values and skills for dealing with socio-economic and political challenges, including cross-cutting issues • Apply life skills in dealing with socio-economic and political challenges, including HIV, globalisation, gender, drug abuse and corruption	Human resource development in Tanzania: 5 hours HIV and AIDS and development: 4 hours Gender and development: 5 hours	• Outline strategies for empowering youth, the disabled and disadvantaged members of the community, including women (one of 6 objectives) • Determine the extent of HIV and AIDS in Tanzania • Assess effectiveness of strategies to alleviate HIV • Point out risk behaviours • Carry out guidance and counselling for effected and affected • Explain concept of gender • Explain relationship between gender issues and development • Analyse policies that are in place for gender equity and equality in Tanzania • Analyse successes and challenges facing women's empowerment in Tanzania	• Case studies, group discussions and presentations, guest speakers • Internet searches, library reading, brainstorming group discussion on how to avoid risk behaviour, guest speakers on guidance, counselling and support • Small group discussions, case studies, use of semantic web and presentations on gender concepts, issues and their impact on development	• Newspapers, newsletters, magazines, reports and modules on development studies in secondary education • Newspapers, magazines, books, research reports, module on development studies • Newspapers, pamphlets, pictures, posters, research reports, module development studies

Table 7.5 (continued)

Course title, objectives and competencies	Topic and time allocated	Topic-specific objectives	Teaching and learning strategies	Teaching and learning resources
Biology academic: • Use biological skills and knowledge to deal positively with cross-cutting issues	HIV and AIDS, sexually transmitted infections (STIs) and STDs: 4 hours Drugs, drug abuse and responsible behaviour: 4 hours	• Explain causes, transmission, symptoms, effects and preventive measures for HIV, STIs and STDs • Outline ways of managing HIV and AIDS, STIs and STDs • Investigate the impact and control of HIV, STIs and STDs • Describe the causes and effects of drug abuse • Suggest preventive and control measures on drugs and drug addiction • Differentiate responsible from irresponsible behaviour	• Brainstorming and presentation, group project to investigate the impact and control of HIV in the neighbouring community, presentation of findings • Guest speaker, role play	• Charts • Pictures, photographs, videos, radio and radio cassettes
English pedagogy: • Integrate cross-cutting issues in the teaching and learning of English				

Table 7.5 (continued)

Course title, objectives and competencies	Topic and time allocated	Topic-specific objectives	Teaching and learning strategies	Teaching and learning resources
Civics pedagogy: • Promote skills for infusing citizenship values, cross-cutting issues, and 'higher' thinking skills	Human rights	• Identify appropriate citizenship and higher thinking to be infused into teaching of human rights • Prepare lesson plans and show how to teach selected subtopics such as human rights	• Peer teaching to demonstrate case studies, role play and small group discussions	
History pedagogy: Infuse cross-cutting issues as they teach				

expected to find this information from other sources. The tutors need to provide some information on HIV and its transmission in order to make the suggested activities more meaningful.

The topic of gender and development is also included in the development studies syllabus and is to be taught over four hours, primarily to raise awareness of the topic. By the end of these sessions the teacher trainees are expected to be able to explain the concept of gender, the relationship between gender and development, and to be able to analyse policies for gender equity and equality and the successes and challenges for women's empowerment in Tanzania. Tutors are expected to use group discussions, case studies, and the semantic web as teaching strategies, and to use newspapers, research reports and the module as resource materials.

The module provides some basic information on the meaning of gender and gender roles in Tanzanian society and on the concepts of equality, equity and women's empowerment. Three activities are recommended, which require trainees to identify gender roles, assess gender equality and equity in their own college, and identify what men can do to promote women's empowerment. They are also asked to reflect on 'how gender discrimination in Tanzania undermines development'. These are context-relevant activities, and they require tutors to be knowledgeable about the topic if they are to support the suggested activities. As with the topic on HIV, so with gender – no content or activity focuses on how future teachers may promote gender-sensitive behaviour amongst young people or maintain gender equality in their own classrooms and schools.

Psychology, guidance and counselling is another compulsory subject in the diploma programme where HIV and gender-related topics are integrated. Within this subject, the topic of social development is assigned eight hours and sexual behaviour is a particular focus in this. Two of the six objectives listed for social development are related to gender and HIV. Trainees are expected to be able to 'argue for and against social cultural practices contributing to gender oppression, discrimination and stereotyping' and to 'demonstrate ways to address the society on gender in relation to HIV and AIDS'. Group study and role plays are recommended as teaching strategies to address 'gender in relation to HIV and AIDS' during this course. Despite much effort, we were unable to obtain all the modules. Hence we cannot say what information is available on this topic and what help tutors may find in the modules to implement the teaching learning strategies recommended in the syllabus.

Amongst the subject specialisation courses, HIV and gender are integrated into biology academic[7] and civics. HIV and sexually transmitted diseases (STDs) are a specific subtopic within the main topic of health and immunity. Approximately four hours are recommended for this subtopic. Student teachers are expected to become able to explain the causes, symptoms, effects and preventive measures for HIV and STDs, outline ways of managing these, and investigate the impact and control of HIV and STDs in their community. The recommended teaching strategies include brainstorming, bringing in guest speakers and organising group projects for investigation. Various teaching resources such as pictures, charts, television, video and radio programmes are recommended. The English and History syllabi list 'infusion of cross-cutting issues' – which would include HIV and gender – as one of several objectives for the courses, but do not follow these up in the recommended teaching, learning strategies or resources.

In summary, while both the certificate and diploma in teaching in Tanzania integrate and infuse HIV and gender in several courses, the purpose of integration remains limited to providing basic knowledge on these topics. For HIV, the primary focus remains on basic knowledge and awareness about the nature of the disease, modes of transmission and strategies for prevention. The syllabi do not include any objectives for influencing trainees' own beliefs and behaviour. Although the certificate course is expected to prepare teachers to teach at the primary level, the syllabi do not include any reference to how HIV and gender issues may be addressed with children at that level. Similarly, the diploma curriculum does not include any objectives or content on how to address these topics with young adults.

Uganda

As mentioned in an earlier section, the policy environment for HIV education in Uganda is quite positive and a number of initiatives have been taken to introduce HIV education in schools, particularly under the Presidential Initiative on the AIDS Strategy for Communication to Youth (PIASCY). However, the country's pre-service teacher education curriculum was last revised in 1994; it does not include HIV or gender education in any significant manner, and neither the general aims of teacher education nor the specific objectives for primary teacher education refer to HIV or gender education directly.

HIV or gender-related content is not explicitly integrated into any of the units within the syllabus for the certificate in primary teacher education in Uganda, although there are several units where there is a possibility of integration (see table 7.6, below). A unit on science and health education, which aims to help student teachers '*acquire the scientific skills necessary for taking informed decisions on issues relating to health, the environment and population*' and '*develop values of responsible parenthood for improved quality of life*', includes some HIV-related content (prevention and transmission and social issues under topics such as human reproduction, human health, traditional medicine and modern drugs. A unit on cultural education also infuses HIV and gender under the topics sex, marriage and family and teaching moral education.

As mentioned earlier, almost all universities in Uganda offer diploma and degree-level courses for teachers' education. However, this report has had to limit its review to the courses offered by Kyambogo University. This university offers a certificate, a diploma and a degree course in early childhood education and development (ECED); a Bachelor of Teacher Education (BTE) in ECED; and a Bachelor of Arts (BA) with education (with options to specialise in either religious studies or English language teaching). Gender and HIV are included minimally in these courses. For example, the syllabus for the certificate in ECED mentions gender under development studies. Another topic, health and nutrition, also refers to HIV and recommends teaching on appropriate nutrition for those suffering from HIV.

The diploma, BEd in ECED and BTE in ECED includes relatively more content on HIV and AIDS. The causes, prevention and care of HIV are included in the recommended content under the topics of child health and family life education. The BA with education courses make no mention of HIV or gender-related issues as topics or subtopics or recommend their infusion. However, as suggested in table 7.7, below, the course on religious studies includes topics where integration and inclusion is possible; for example, under the topics: sex, marriage, family life, life and death issues,

Table 7.6 Integration of HIV and gender into subject syllabus in primary teacher education curriculum in Uganda

Subject	Key objectives	Topic content/units	Suggested teaching methods	Mention and integration of HIV and gender
Professional education studies (PES): 195 hours over course, i.e. 5 hours per week	• Acquisition of specialist knowledge • Development of deeper insight into the principles behind teaching methods • Equip students with techniques for teaching young children • Skills to interpret, implement and evaluate syllabus • Develop creative abilities	• Human growth and development • Curriculum development in primary schools • Learning in the primary school • General methods and strategies of teaching • Early childhood education and instruction • Managing of instruction in middle and upper primary classes • Classroom communication and instruction aids • Development of education in Uganda • The development of Uganda's formal education system • Teaching study skills in the primary school • Guidance and counselling in primary schools	• Conventional teaching methods • Dramatisation/group methods • Role playing • Peer teaching • Discussion • Brainstorming • Field trips	The PES course has 16 units, each with its own objectives. Neither HIV nor gender is mentioned in any of these objectives. HIV is not mentioned in the PES course content. Gender is taught under the following units: • Development of education in Uganda: female education is discussed under topic imbalances in the education system HIV and gender are also inferred in the following units: • Guidance and counselling • Sociological issues in primary education • School and community mobilisation Explicit mention and integration of HIV is possible in the following units:

Table 7.6 (continued)

Subject	Key objectives	Topic content/ units	Suggested teaching methods	Mention and integration of HIV and gender
Professional education studies (PES): (continued)		• Educational evaluation • School administration, management and planning • Managing resources in primary schools • Sociological issues in primary schools • Application of philosophy in education		• Human growth and development School administration, management and planning Curriculum development in primary schools • Early childhood education and instruction
English language with literature: 216 hours over course, i.e. 4 hours a week	• Express themselves in simple, correct oral and written English and likewise be able to teach the same to their pupils in primary schools • Practice the appropriate methods and techniques of teaching English language with literature effectively • Acquire the necessary effective reading and writing skills, which they can utilise for their personal study and also later pass on to pupils	• Introduction to teaching primary English • Approaches to teaching primary English • Language acquisition young children • Teaching oral English in lower primary classes • Creativity in the teaching of oral skills • Teaching reading in primary school • Teaching writing at primary level • Controlled, guided and free composition	• Lectures • Projects • Audio-visual aids • Micro-teaching	The English course has 16 units, each with its own objectives. Neither HIV nor gender is mentioned in any of these objectives Mention and integration of HIV and gender would apply in the following units: • Creativity in the teaching of oral skills • Simple literature in drama and poetry

Table 7.6 (continued)

Subject	Key objectives	Topic content/units	Suggested teaching methods	Mention and integration of HIV and gender
English language with literature (continued)	• Practice functional and creative writing skills, supported by wide and selective reading • Identify the basic characteristic needs and underlying psychology of individual pupils so they can be helped accordingly • Become acquainted with the various approaches, methods and techniques of teaching the four basic language skills at lower, middle and upper primary levels • Practice the techniques of organisation and improvisation at lower, middle and upper primary levels • Handle and guide learners to study literature books in primary schools	• Language improvement principles and practice of teaching • Basic principles of teaching reading • Developing fluency and comprehension in reading • Note taking and summary writing • Functional and creative writing • Teaching writing to beginners • Improvisation in English language teaching • Techniques in writing		

Table 7.6 (continued)

Subject	Key objectives	Topic content/units	Suggested teaching methods	Mention and integration of HIV and gender
English language with literature (continued)	• Select and use appropriate improvisation techniques for teaching various language aspects in the primary school • Outline details of content of language teaching materials at each of the three levels of the primary school system • Design and use appropriate teaching language games at the various levels			
Social studies: 216 hours over course, i.e. 4 hours a week	• Knowledge acquisition, including basic principles of social studies • Acquisition of manipulative and social skills • Appreciative attitudes and values, including the identification of problems in teaching and learning, social studies and solutions to them	• Introduction to social studies • Teaching and learning social studies • People's activities and the environment • Our local environment • Introduction to Uganda • Development of Uganda into a state • Post-independence developments and challenges	• Learner-centred approaches • Experiential learning • Inter-and multi-disciplinary approaches • Multi-media • Peer teaching • Projects	The social studies course has 14 units, each with its own objectives. Neither HIV nor gender is mentioned in any of these objectives. The course comprises units on history and geography. Topics focus on self, family, home, school, neighbourhood, nations and the world, but no mention is made of HIV or gender. HIV and gender would apply in the following units:

Table 7.6 (continued)

Subject	Key objectives	Topic content/units	Suggested teaching methods	Mention and integration of HIV and gender
Social studies (continued)		• Map work and photo-graphic interpretation • East Africa: physical environment and natural resources • East Africa: the people, colonialism and independence • Africa: physical environment and people • Africa: early empires, colonisation and independence • The world • International co-operation and the search for peace		• People's activities and the environment • Post-independence developments and challenges
Science with health education: 216 hours over course, i.e. 4 hours a week	• Develop positive attitudes towards science, including the promotion of health and protection of the environment • Acquire basic understanding and knowledge of science and health through of process skills	• Introduction to teaching primary science • Energy resources • Physical properties of materials • Air, water and sanitation • Raw materials and chemical products	• Learner-centred approaches • Field trips • Individual research • Experimentation • Case studies • Report writing	The science with health course has 17 units, each with its own objectives. Neither HIV nor gender is mentioned in any of these objectives, but HIV content is found in the units below: • Human bones, muscle and circulatory systems: HIV is

Table 7.6 (continued)

Subject	Key objectives	Topic content/units	Suggested teaching methods	Mention and integration of HIV and gender
Science with health education: (continued)	• Solve problems of a scientific and technological nature • Improve individual teaching of science objectives by innovative learning activities • Analyse interaction between population and environment • Develop awareness of the effect of population on quality of the individual, the family, the community, the nation, the world • Acquire the scientific skills necessary for taking informed decisions on issues relating to health, the environment and population • Acquire communication skills for sharing important scientific information in order to improve the quality of life • Develop values of responsible parenthood for improved quality of life	• Machines • Electricity and magnetism • Sound and light • Earth and space • Introduction to the environment • Introduction to the human body • Human bones, muscle and circulatory systems • Systems that process air, water and control body processes • Human reproduction • Human health • Traditional medicine and modern drugs	• Dramatisation	taught as a disease of the blood (p. 42) • Systems that process air, water and food: content covers signs and symptoms of HIV as a disease, definitions of HIV and AIDS, methods of HIV transmission, science behind HIV virus infection (pp. 44-45) • Human reproduction: content covers HIV as an epidemic, HIV in sex education, care of the reproductive system in males and females (pp. 112, 119, 133) • Human health: content covers HIV as a communicable disease and a sexually transmitted disease (pp. 141, 156) • Traditional medicine and modern drugs: HIV transmission is covered under a topic on the administration of traditional medicine (p. 187)

Table 7.6 (continued)

Subject	Key objectives	Topic content/units	Suggested teaching methods	Mention and integration of HIV and gender
Mathematics: 216 hours over course, i.e. 4 hours a week		• Pre-mathematical activities and learning theories • Organising mathematics lessons • Organising mathematics classrooms • Numeration systems and place values • Teaching addition and subtraction of whole numbers • Teaching multiplication and division of whole numbers • Extending the number system • Rational numbers • Decimal fractions • Ration, proportion and percentage • Easy methods of computation • Set concepts • Relations and functions	• Individual work • Group work • Dramatisation • Experimentation	The mathematics course has 21 units, each with its own objectives. Neither HIV nor gender is mentioned in any of these objectives. The content does not mention HIV or gender anywhere, although it would apply in the following topics: • Statistics • Organising the mathematics classroom

Table 7.6 (continued)

Subject	Key objectives	Topic content/ units	Suggested teaching methods	Mention and integration of HIV and gender
		• Algebra • Linear measures • Mass, weight and capacity • Temperature, time and money • Geometry 1 • Geometry 2 • Statistics • Probability		
Cultural education: 216 hours over course, i.e. 4 hours a week	• Cultural education deliberately attempts to cater for traditional cultures, norms and values that society identifies itself through; the systemic study and appreciation of aesthetic values of arts and crafts, music and dance; ethical values in moral education; and physical values in physical education	• Art appreciation • Drawing, painting and graphic design • Modelling and sculpture • Fabric design • Construction and assembly • Teaching art and craft in the primary school • Music development in Uganda • Major periods in the development of Western music • Rhythm, pitch, scales and key signatures		The cultural education course has four sections and 24 units covering arts and crafts, music education, moral education and physical education. Each section has 6 units, each with its own objectives. Neither HIV nor gender is mentioned in any of these objectives, but HIV content is found in the unit below: Moral education: • Sex, marriage and family – makes reference to HIV and gender in the following topic areas covering the concept of

Table 7.6 (continued)

Subject	Key objectives	Topic content/units	Suggested teaching methods	Mention and integration of HIV and gender
Cultural education (continued)		• Musical terms and signs, time form and aural training • Background to the study of morals • Religion and morality • Character building in contemporary society • Sex, marriage and family • Leadership • Human beings and resource management • Teaching moral education • Acquisition of motor skills and methods of teaching physical education • Build up games • Gymnastics • Athletics • Netball • Soccer		sex and sexuality, gender balance, proper use of sex, sex abuse and misuse, choosing a marriage partner, marriage, family life, separation and divorce (pp. 96–123) • Teaching moral education in the primary school – refers to HIV in the context of need for moral education in the primary school curriculum (pp. 183–193)

work and leisure, contemporary ethical problems, the role of women and society, polygamy, property, slavery and war, and the status of women in Islam. Topics such as child rights, family life and issues of development included in the other courses also offer possibilities for inclusion of HIV and gender-related issues, although these are not mentioned specifically in the syllabi.

As apparent from the above description, gender and HIV education is only minimally integrated into the current teacher education curriculum documents in Uganda. However, teaching and learning materials for gender and HIV education have been developed and distributed to all primary teachers' colleges in the country, primarily under the Presidential Initiative on the AIDS Strategy for Communication to Youth (PIASCY). These materials include students' learning materials, as well as handbooks for teachers (see table 7.8, below). The teachers' handbooks are entitled *Helping children to stay safe*. There are two volumes, one for primary years 3 and 4 and a second for primary years 5 and 6. These volumes aim to provide teachers with content knowledge and skills for teaching children about sexuality, reproductive health, sexually transmitted diseases, HIV and AIDS, children's rights and responsibilities and life skills. Most importantly, they guide teachers on how to teach children about sexuality and to help them to choose to abstain. The objectives of the second volume (for teachers teaching primary 5 and 6) are more specific about increasing and sustaining HIV and AIDS education for school-going children, and increasing the capacity of parents and teachers to engage in constructive debates with young people on HIV. The handbooks guide teachers on how to use 'interactive activities' in class, such as pair and group work, songs and stories, as well as awareness raising activities during assembly. The design of these materials is user-friendly and they can be used in college and school assemblies to spread strong HIV messages, on abstinence, stigmatisation and inclusiveness, awareness and sensitisation in classrooms, and the 'talking compound' (schools display HIV and health messages in their compounds, referred to a 'talking compound', as part of the awareness campaign).

Similarly, two teachers' handbooks on gender and education have been developed. The first (Mlama, Marema and Makoye, 2005) published by the Forum for African Women Educationalists (FAWE), aims at helping teachers become gender responsive in their lesson planning, in the use of language

Table 7.7 Integration of HIV and gender into teacher education courses at university in Uganda

Course	Key objectives	Topic content	Suggested teaching methods	Mention and integration of HIV and gender
Certificate in early childhood education and development (ECED)	Produce ECED teachers who will apply knowledge, skills, values and attitudes to competently address the learning needs of children in Uganda during their early years of development	• Knowledge of ECED • Professional studies • Educational technology • Language theory • Methods and approaches to teaching in ECED • Early childhood education and development • Child study • Mathematics theory • School practice • Administration and management • Child health and nutrition • Language education in ECED • Mathematics education in ECED • ICT • Cultural education • Development studies • Special needs education • School practice	• Lectures • Projects • Practice	• Mention of gender is made in development studies. Otherwise, it can be inferred in professional studies, child-friendly centres/ schools and child study • HIV is mentioned in child health and nutrition as a disease requiring special nutrition

Table 7.7 (continued)

Course	Key objectives	Topic content	Suggested teaching methods	Mention and integration of HIV and gender
Diploma in early childhood education and development (ECED)	Produce ECED teachers who will apply knowledge, skills, values and attitudes to competently address the learning needs of children in Uganda during their early years of development	• Knowledge of ECED • Child health and nutrition • Children's rights and responsibilities • Professional studies • Educational technology • Play as an avenue for learning • Methods and approaches to teaching • ECED curricula • Community involvement • School practice • Assessment and evaluation • Administration and management • Language in ECED • Mathematics education in ECED • Science education in ECED • Cultural education • ICT • Business skills • Environmental education • Professional education in ECED • Special needs education	• Lectures • Research project • Practice	• Gender coverage could be inferred in social development, children's rights and responsibilities; play as an avenue for learning • HIV is mentioned in child health and nutrition; coverage can be inferred in children's rights and responsibilities and professional studies

Table 7.7 (continued)

Course	Key objectives	Topic content	Suggested teaching methods	Mention and integration of HIV and gender
Bachelor of early childhood education and development (ECED)	Equip ECED teachers with quality knowledge, skills, values and attitudes necessary to competently address the learning needs of young children in Uganda during their early years of learning from 0–8 years	• Introduction to early childhood • Child growth, development and rearing practices • Child health • Child nutrition • Methods and approaches to teaching young children • Child study in ECED • ECED curricula • Play in ECED • Language development and literacy • Science education in ECED • Mathematics education in ECED • Cultural values and practices in ECED • Administration and management of early childhood institutions • ICT in ECED • Business skills and entrepreneurship	• Lectures • Research project • School practice	• Gender coverage could be inferred under domestic violence and its influence on child development; there is explicit mention of gender equality and equity, family issues and family life education in early childhood education • HIV is mentioned in child health; the focus is causes, prevention and care of HIV and AIDS patients

Table 7.7 (continued)

Course	Key objectives	Topic content	Suggested teaching methods	Mention and integration of HIV and gender
Bachelor of early childhood education and development (ECED) (continued)		• Research in ECED • Assessment and evaluation in ECED • Special needs education in ECED • Community education and involvement in ECED • Family issues and family life in ECD • Contemporary issues in ECD • School practice • Research report		
Bachelor of Teacher Education in early childhood education and development (ECED)	Equip tutors with quality knowledge, skills and attitudes necessary to competently address the learning needs of early childhood education students in teacher education institutions		• Lectures • Practice	• Gender coverage could be inferred in special needs education in early childhood education under inclusive education, family issues and family life education in early childhood education • Gender equality and equity are explicitly mentioned under family issues and family life education in early childhood education • HIV is mentioned in child health and nutrition; the focus is causes, prevention and care of HIV and AIDS patients

Table 7.7 (continued)

Course	Key objectives	Topic content	Suggested teaching methods	Mention and integration of HIV and gender
Bachelor of Arts in Education (religious studies)	No objectives given	• Phenomenology of religion • Introduction to ethics 1 and 11 • African traditional religions • Introduction to *The Bible*/Islam • Sociology of religion • *The Old Testament* • Systematic theology • Theology and traditions of Islam • Philosophy of religion • History of religion in Uganda • Methods • *The New Testament* • World religions	• Lectures • Research project	• The Bachelor of Arts in Education (religious studies) syllabus makes no mention of gender, but coverage is inferred in topics on sex, marriage, family life, issues of life and death; work and leisure taught under 'Introduction to ethics 1: contemporary ethical problems' • Gender coverage possible in the role of women and society, marriage, polygamy, property, slavery and war taught under 'the society'. Also in the topic status of women in Islam under 'Basic teaching of the *Qur'an*' • There is no mention of HIV, although coverage could be inferred within the topics human dignity, human rights and freedom, duty and responsibility, justice, the state and the citizen under 'Social ethics and social development'

Table 7.7 (continued)

Course	Key objectives	Topic content	Suggested teaching methods	Mention and integration of HIV and gender
Bachelor of Arts in Education (English language teaching)	No objectives given	A selection of topics include: • Introduction to the study of language • The receptive skills of communication • Language analysis and communication • The structure of English • English phonetics and phonology • Language acquisition • Functional varieties of English • Socio-linguistics • Language policies • Discourse analysis • Introduction to literature • East African literature • African literature • Language and style	• Lectures	• There is no mention of HIV or gender, although it could be taught within language use in relation to sociological variables, which falls under 'Socio-linguistics'; both could also be integrated in discourse analysis • Gender coverage possible in feminism under 'Modern critical approaches and language acquisition'

Table 7.7 (continued)

Course	Key objectives	Topic content	Suggested teaching methods	Mention and integration of HIV and gender
Bachelor of Arts in Education (English literature)	• Understanding of what literature is • Appreciation of literary criticism • Knowledge and skills to teach literature at all levels of secondary education	A selection of topics include: • Introduction to literature • East African literature • Modes of criticism • Oral literature • Poetry • Theatre arts • Creative writing • Literature teaching methodology • Classical literature	• Lecture • Research report in English language teaching (ELT)	• The Bachelor of Arts in Education (English literature) syllabus allows coverage of gender in the feminist approach, feminism and literature and feminist literary theory and criticism taught under 'Modes of criticism: critical concepts and approaches' • There is no mention or implication of coverage of HIV, though books on this theme could be included among recommended texts for the course

in the class and in classroom management and to address issues, such as sexual harassment, which affect gender relations in the classroom but which are not addressed in pre-service training. The second handbook (REPLICA, 2006) is a '*teaching resource for teachers, school managers, service providers and the community for guiding and mobilising support for promotion of girls' education*'; it provides gender responsive strategies for whole school improvement.

These materials provide clear guidance on how to integrate HIV and gender into teaching, although some of the content is pitched at a level which may not be appropriate for very young children. They are meant for in-service teacher guidance and support, and have been used to provide in-service training to almost all primary teachers in Uganda and to selected tutors from teacher education colleges. It is expected that these materials will used in pre-service training. However, as is evident from the descriptions in the various syllabi, no space has been created within the country's current curriculum for integrating HIV or gender education.

Table 7.8 HIV and gender material used in primary teacher education in Uganda

Book	Key objectives	Teaching methods suggested	Content	Mention and integration of HIV and gender
Helping Pupils To Stay Safe: A Handbook for Teachers, pp. 3–4 (PIASCY First Edition)	• Helping pupils to stay safe	• Interactive activities, e.g. pair and group work • Story telling • Dramatisation	• How to pass on information about sexuality to children • Ethics, morals and cultural values • Reproductive health • Gender, children's rights and responsibilities • Life skills • HIV and AIDS • Sexually transmitted infections • Guidance and counselling • Messages for assemblies, clubs and classes	• The entire focus of the book is HIV and AIDS. The book has detailed content on the subject and useful teaching tips and activities for teachers. However, in some sections the content is somewhat dense and pitched above the cognitive level of development of 9 to 10 year olds. • The poem suggested for teaching on sexually transmitted infections (p. 84) is easy to learn and recite, but in terms of content can 9–10 year olds understand the biology of the disease or even relate it to their underdeveloped reproductive bodies? The poem makes mention of infections in the vagina and penis oozing with pus. The poem is unlikely to impact on children of this age group, because they may not understand the issues discussed in the poem. • The section on myths about menstruation and sex (p. 38) is also pitched beyond the level of 9–10 year olds, many of whom may not have had the onset of menses or understand discourse related to sex and sexuality.

Table 7.8 (continued)

Book	Key objectives	Teaching methods suggested	Content	Mention and integration of HIV and gender
Helping Pupils To Stay Safe: A Handbook for Teachers, pp. 5–7 (PIASCY First Edition)	• To increase and sustain HIV education for school-going children • To increase the capacity of parents and teachers to engage in constructive deliberations with young people on HIV and AIDS	• Interactive activities, e.g. pair and group work • Story telling • Songs and poetry	• Helping pupils to choose and abstain • Ethics, morals and cultural values • Teaching reproductive health and HIV • Understanding HIV and AIDS in Uganda • Gender, children's rights and responsibilities • Reproductive health • STIs, HIV and AIDS • Life skills • Guidance and counselling • Messages for assemblies, clubs and classes	• The entire focus of the book is HIV and AIDS. The book has detailed content on the subject and useful teaching tips and activities for teachers. • The content integrates HIV and AIDS with gender, gender roles, children's rights, reproductive rights and gender violence. The book covers HIV testing, abstinence, faithfulness, condom use and pregnancy.

Table 7.8 (continued)

Book	Key objectives	Teaching methods suggested	Content	Mention and integration of HIV and gender
Gender responsive pedagogy: A teachers' handbook	• To make gender responsive in the teaching process, such as lesson planning, teaching and learning materials, language use in the classroom, classroom set up and class-room interaction • To delve into certain issues which greatly affect gender relations in the classrooms, but which are rarely if ever tackled in pre-service training	• Not explicitly indicated, but group work, interactive discussions and role modelling are inferred	• What is 'gender responsive pedagogy' • Gender responsive lesson planning • Gender responsive teaching and learning materials • Gender responsive language use in classrooms • Gender responsive classroom set up • Gender responsive management of sexual maturation • Sexual harassment • Supportive gender responsive school management systems	• The entire focus of the book is on gender and it is specifically intended to make teachers and learners gender aware and responsive in teaching and learning processes, as well as in the support given and attitudes held.

Table 7.8 (continued)

Book	Key objectives	Teaching methods suggested	Content	Mention and integration of HIV and gender
The basics promotion of girls' education: A handbook for guiding action and mobilising support	• A teaching resource for teachers, school managers, service providers and the community for guiding and mobilising support for the promotion of girls' education	• Case studies • Role play and skits • Discussions • Record keeping	• Gender responsive teaching and teachers • Gender responsive school managers • Sensitising and mobilising communities towards becoming gender responsive	• The focus of the book is gender. The book advocates for whole school and whole community gender aware and gender responsive strategies.

Chapter 8

Curriculum in Practice

As described above, pre-service teacher training curricula across the three East African countries considered in this report include some HIV and gender-related content in various subjects and units, particularly science, civics, social studies, development studies and religious education. The principals and tutors interviewed were aware of the curriculum and its recommendations, as demonstrated in the following quotes from interviewers' notes:

> *'In all five colleges visited, trainees and tutors said that HIV and AIDS and gender is infused and integrated in the official curriculum. A tutor defined infusion as including HIV and gender issues while teaching a topic which includes neither HIV nor gender content. As for integration, a science tutor said this is the inclusion of gender and HIV in a topic that has related content, like reproductive health education'.*
>
> (From an interviewer's notes on interviews at teachers' colleges in Kenya)

> *'Tutors and students were aware that HIV and gender are integrated in the syllabi of the various subjects in the certificate and diploma courses'.*
>
> (From an interviewer's notes on interviews in teachers' colleges in Tanzania)

> *'HIV and AIDS is included in the science syllabus. In other subjects, teachers are supposed to integrate it. For example, in English language, they can include it in debates and comprehension passage. In music, dance and drama, they can compose songs and perform skits on an HIV theme. In the foundation of education subject, a tutor can integrate HIV and AIDS education when teaching life skills. But in all these subjects, HIV and AIDS education is not stated as a topic or a subtopic'.*
>
> (Tutor at a primary teachers' college [PTC] in Uganda)

This chapter describes and discusses the implementation of HIV and gender-related objectives and content of the curricula into the classrooms of teacher education colleges in Kenya, Tanzania and Uganda. In particular, it describes the amount of classroom time spent on these topics, the teaching approaches used, and the teaching and learning materials available and used in the sample colleges in each country.

Kenya

Tutors in Kenyan teacher training colleges seemed to spend very little classroom time on teaching content or skills related to HIV education. According to one tutor, '*It is really hard to say how much time I spent. Sometimes I mention HIV and gender issues during their normal lessons in a minute or two. I could say not much time is given ... a total of 4 to 5 hours for the entire two year course*'. Other tutors interviewed gave similar descriptions, and explained that one of the main reasons for this situation was that HIV and gender-related content was an 'add on' to an already full syllabus for particular subjects, rather than its being integrated with adequate time allocated for teaching. A mathematics tutor explained:

> '*In mathematics, for example, it is mentioned only in the context of reduced population numbers: if HIV and AIDS attacked a population and it dropped by a given percentage, and this was the population, what will be the new population of that town or that region. But we don't have any specific time set aside for teaching HIV and AIDS. It is up to you as the teacher to come up with a question that deals with it. But it is there in the syllabus that this is supposed to be integrated in the subject*'.

Tutors emphasised that '*HIV and AIDS [education] should not be an additional responsibility*'; and most insisted that these topics '*should be taught as a separate subject and be given one hour. This is because when we infuse and integrate, a tutor may miss out or forget to mention the expected content*'. Tutors also reported that even if they had the time to teach, the syllabus lacks detailed content. Several tutors agreed on this and suggested that '*The syllabus should be revised so that these topics can go deeper, because what we have is just touching a bit, they are not going deep*'.

Kenya's curriculum documents suggest integration of topics as well as a recommended list of participatory teaching strategies. However, it seems that the primary method of teaching at the training colleges is the transmission of information through lectures; participatory approaches seemed to be used rarely. The science tutor at one college, for example, reported that he used science textbooks containing information on HIV and AIDS to give lectures, which students were to note. A trainee described her class as follows: '*We wrote notes on different ways of controlling HIV and AIDS*'.

In some instances, tutors used demonstration or assigned 'project work'; however, these were either teacher-centred or unguided. For example, a trainee described a class as follows: '*The tutor showed us two beakers containing a colourless liquid. We were asked to compare the two. They were the same, but when the tutor added an indicator to both the solutions, one turned red while the other one remained colourless. This was an illustration that you cannot know if somebody is positive by merely looking at them ... you have to carry out a test*'. However, further description of the class sessions suggested that tutors did not encourage class interaction, nor did they make their teaching responsive to the trainees' needs; in fact, students' questions were discomforting for the tutors. One tutor expressed his frustration: '*How can I teach people who are not interested in what I am teaching, but just want to ask many questions*'. Other tutors also mentioned using project work. However, these mostly required students to find answers to questions regarding transmission and prevention of HIV, or reasons why HIV was a burden on society, and then to come back with a report. Tutors did not seem to provide any guidance or direct effective classroom discussion on the information students brought to class. The 'project work' was attractive to teachers, because they did not have to deal directly with what they referred to as 'sensitive topics' in class. As one tutor explained:

> *If they [students] have projects and all these explanations from the projects and the samples from [them], actually it's a good method of teaching because people will learn. People might not want to hear, they want to shy off. When they are learning they are observing and seeing*'. (Tutor)

According to another tutor:

> '*HIV and AIDS is not as serious [seriously embarrassing or sensitive] as teaching reproductive organs, because that one talks about the private things deeply. But this one [i.e. HIV and AIDS] there are other areas like causes* and *how to prevent it, which does not deeply look at other sources [other than sex]*

> *of transmission. So, it does not have that difficulty, but however, sometimes there are people who do not want to hear about it. They almost break their ears because it is something which is vulnerable to them'.* (Tutor)

Some tutors seemed to use HIV and gender-related content to, as one student put it and others agreed, *'flavour a dull lecture'*. *'They use HIV and AIDS and gender issues as jokes to rekindle interest in the lesson. As soon as the tutors get the trainees' attention, they revert back to the carrier subject matter, without exhaustively addressing the HIV or gender issue they had raised'*. According to the trainees, this attitude belittles HIV and gender-related content and suggests that it is non-serious and non-essential knowledge.

Trainees were dissatisfied with the teaching and the information provided in class and in books, because these did not help them address challenges they faced in their personal lives or those they may face in their professional lives as teachers. For example, female students at one college were particularly concerned with the stigma associated with condom use. A student expressed her fears of rejection: *'If my boyfriend finds me with a condom, he may think that I am sleeping with other men'*. Others were worried about their preparedness to teach: *'We talk about HIV and AIDS, but there are no text books with all the information one can use. What will I use when I am in my class?'*

Tutors and trainees in all colleges in the Kenyan sample complained about the lack of relevant and effective teaching learning materials available to them on HIV and AIDS education. Textbooks were the primary and most often the only resource available and used for teaching and learning all subjects; yet only the science textbook had any content on HIV and AIDS. Even when material was available, as it was in at least one college visited, this was not accessed by the tutors or trainees, but was stored in a room. At one college which was participating in an HIV education-related project and had considerable material available, the HIV co-ordinator claimed that teachers *'are normally free to come here [to his office] and then they get that information, we tell them what we know'*. However, he also complained about the lack of relevant materials for teacher education:

> *'Actually there is no information at all at any college. We do not have any specific [material related to HIV and AIDS], like here in the college, I don't think we have any specific books for that. They [materials for teaching HIV*

and AIDS] are not there, there aren't [any]. So as much as the ministry has infused this topic, they have not come up with any, any particular material that could be, say, specific, that could be useful. They are not there'.

Teacher trainees also complained that most topics and information in the curricula, books and other materials were repetitive and did not meet their needs for new and more detailed knowledge. According to one trainee:

'We have learnt this stuff in high school. Things like definition, transmission and prevention was all taught in school and they are repeated here. We just repeat them here for exams. We should be learning more detailed stuff, like why are some couples positive yet the partner remains negative?'

(Trainee in a focus group discussion)

Tutors were similarly dissatisfied, as reflected in the following quote from a tutor who said:

'We don't have a particular book that is on HIV and AIDS. We have a creative book or PE book, we should have a HIV book, so that everything is there. A teacher is supposed to relate everything from the title. What we have does not expose the teacher to everything, he is just limited.'

Both tutors and trainees in Kenya believed that tutors needed better preparation to implement HIV education in general, and the integrated curriculum in particular. When asked if they found teaching HIV and gender easy or challenging, tutors gave different responses. Those who had received some training under the Centre for British Teachers (CfBT) programme and those who had specialised in and taught science seemed to feel more prepared to teach HIV in class. One CfBT-trained tutor expressed his confidence and said, *'I have information ... for people without information; it can be very difficult, like when you talk about the infection, progression from HIV to AIDS. Sometimes it can be very technical if you do not have the information'*. Science tutors also felt that they were able to teach HIV, because they possessed scientific knowledge. Tutors of other subjects, such as social studies, felt more challenged and less prepared to integrate HIV education into their subject lessons. The view that HIV education is about transmission of scientific knowledge is reflected in the curriculum, classroom teaching practice and in the tutors' own assessments of their capacity to teach.

As described above, very little class time is spent on HIV education in the regular timetable. However, some colleges had organised short HIV-awareness sessions or workshops outside of the regular timetable. In one college, for example, an awareness workshop is usually held towards the end of the pre-service training programme. At another college, such workshops are conducted as part of the orientation programme for newly enrolled students at the beginning of the academic year. A tutor who facilitated these workshops described them as '*Sensitisation sessions for trainees to protect them from infection and to make them realise that if you live with those already with it … you are either infected or affected*'. The content of the workshops includes 'stigma and discrimination, behaviour change, communication approaches, sexuality and relationships, HIV and AIDS workplace challenges and positive living'. The workshops are about making tutors aware of how to protect themselves and how to deal with HIV and AIDS in their personal lives and in the workplace. However, there is no attempt to raise awareness about their role as teachers responsible for providing HIV and AIDS education to children and young adults in their workplace, which is the school.

The above description of the implementation of the curriculum in the area of HIV suggests that in primary teacher training colleges in Kenya, HIV is taught as a topic mainly under science. It is either mentioned fleetingly or ignored altogether in teaching other subjects, even when included in the syllabus. Moreover, HIV education is perceived as an additional responsibility and added content to already full syllabi for various subjects. Tutors know that they are expected to integrate the issue, but lack time to do so, have non-serious attitudes, lack teaching materials and lack expertise and adequate preparation – all of which contribute to a reluctance to translate and implement the curriculum effectively in classrooms in teacher education colleges.

In Kenya, pre-service training for potential secondary school teachers is provided at university. At the one university in our sample, HIV education is taught as a separate, examinable and compulsory course comprising 35 hours of face-to-face teaching, which is offered during a semester in the first academic year of all teacher-training programmes offered by the university. Two tutors are assigned to teach this subject. These tutors were very enthusiastic about teaching the course and used a course plan and teaching materials (a book) they had themselves developed in co-operation with medical doctors. All trainees interviewed reported that the HIV education classes were held regularly and the tutors followed the course outlines. However, some trainees suggested that they needed more experiential learning, where they would work with those affected by and infected with HIV and AIDS. A few students, members of the university health club, had had further training on peer counselling and community service. The members of this group were confident and felt well prepared to teach HIV education in schools.

Although gender is included as a cross-cutting issue in Kenya's primary and secondary teacher training curriculum and interviewees said that the issue was integrated, we could not obtain information on how often it was taught or what was taught. This lack of information and evidence suggests that gender education is not integrated into the actual teaching of any of the subjects in the primary teacher training colleges or into the university pre-service programme for secondary school teachers.

Tanzania

As in Kenya, tutors and trainees in our sample colleges in Tanzania were aware of HIV and gender being integrated into the syllabi of various subjects in the certificate and diploma programmes; however, it was difficult to get a sense of exactly how much class time is actually spent on these topics. Students from the same college gave very different responses ranging from '*No time spent*' to '*Once every week*'. It seemed that tutors do follow the syllabus and spend more time on the topic of HIV in the science and civics classes for diploma students; some reported '*up to four periods of 45 minutes each*'. Yet trainees who do not specialise in these subjects may not spend any class time on the issues. In other subjects where HIV and gender are subtopics or expected to be infused, tutors may ignore them. One tutor explained that since '*Time [to spend on teaching these topics] is not indicated [in the syllabus], it is left to the tutor to look at the content and allocate time…*'.

HIV education in teacher training colleges comprised transmission of basic knowledge about cause, prevention and effects of HIV, primarily through using lectures and the 'question/answer' method. Some tutors reported engaging students in group discussions around questions assigned by the tutor, or group tasks (similar to project work in Kenya) where trainees were asked to find information on assigned questions and then present their answers to the class. The assigned questions asked about definitions of HIV and AIDS, modes of transmission and prevention. Only one tutor and his students reported doing a role play on the traditional circumcision ceremony. However, the learning objectives for this activity were not apparent to them. Some tutors said that they would like to invite religious leaders and doctors as guest speakers to their classrooms, but none had done so.

The following quotes from students illustrate common teaching practices in teacher training colleges in Tanzania's colleges:

> *'In the HIV and AIDS class, the teacher asked us questions about what HIV is, causes and prevention and then our role was to respond to the questions by explaining'.*
>
> (Student describing the special session on HIV and AIDS)

> *[In the Biology class] I participated in a group discussion where the teacher used more time to organise groups to discuss questions concerning HIV and AIDS. Teachers gave us guidelines for discussion. For instance [he asked us] to describe the structure of virus, causes of HIV and AIDS and how they duplicate, how difficult it is to kill the virus [in a microbiology course]. Teachers also taught us how HIV and AIDS is a pandemic'.*

> *'I taught HIV and AIDS education on traditional practices like initiation ceremonies, whereby people tend to share instruments (like scissors, blades and knives) during circumcision. These practices can lead to infection and transmission of the virus. I organised students in groups to play actions, for example they acted on traditional ceremonies like circumcisions. ... I taught my students about biological changes in humans; these will help them understand their students during teaching in schools'.*

> *'In guidance and counselling, I usually organise sessions (about 30 minutes) with class leaders (peer educators.) I give them topics to educate their colleagues'.*

> *'I participated in the upgrading in-service from grade B to grade A, where teachers were required to prepare posters about HIV and AIDS. We guided teachers to mention [the] effects [of] HIV and AIDS on the communities they come from'.*

It was clear from the interviews that tutors' understanding of HIV education is often superficial, and teaching tends to focus on reviewing basic knowledge about transmission and prevention. Some tutors thought that HIV was easy to teach as a topic because trainee teachers '*are already aware of the disease and can answer basic questions about prevention*'. However, other tutors thought that it was hard to teach, primarily because it offended prior beliefs:

> *'[It is] hard to teach because you need to be open to the trainees when teaching HIV and AIDS topics. Sometimes it is difficult to convince them with their beliefs [religious and traditional]; some trainees feel shy when I mention sexual parts.'*

Trainee teachers and tutors recognised the importance HIV education for future teachers and their students in schools, but their understanding of the purpose of this education was limited to awareness raising and acquiring basic 'scientific' knowledge. They did not expect HIV education to develop life skills or to bring about life-long changes in behaviour. In the trainees' words, the purpose of HIV education in schools is: '*to guide and advise students on the use of condoms* ...'; '*[to] educate students on the meaning of transmission and prevention*'; '*[and to] engage children in a lot of activities, so as to occupy them and avoid sexual behaviour*'. ... '*The need for teaching HIV and AIDS is due to the fact that at that level students are easily infected through sharing food and various things*'. Only one tutor in our sample seemed dissatisfied with the syllabus and thought that the focus should not be transmission of content knowledge and the objectives of teaching. '*What is important is to focus on change in behaviour*', he said.

The researchers saw no teaching learning materials for gender and/or HIV education in the sample colleges, although tutors and trainees reported that they used modules prepared by the Tanzania Institute of Education (reviewed in the last section), pamphlets on HIV received from Tanzania Commission for AIDS [TACAIDS] and materials downloaded from the Internet. Modules were available in some, though not all, colleges and there was no way of verifying other materials because they were not readily available for us to share. Some tutors used the biology book prescribed for A-level and the Bachelor of Science (BSc) courses. Most trainees were dissatisfied with materials, which were either not available or included too little information, or were available but in bulky and unattractive books that did not prepare them to work with children and young people in schools:

> *'In our college surroundings you can see no posters, even in our classes. [We could learn better] if we could have materials like CDs instead of depending on lecturers; in teaching HIV and AIDS there was no poster used'.*
>
> (Trainee)

Tutors were dissatisfied with their preparation to teach, and their students said that they would like to learn more than what they already knew about the topic:

> *'Some topics enlightened me on HIV and AIDS, but I found some topics confusing and unclear, like the source of HIV and AIDS. Some people say that the origin of HIV is from gays. Therefore you cannot get [the] real source, so it is difficult to convince students on this. I do not have answers for my [future] students [in schools] on this and I will teach as I am taught'.*
>
> (Trainee)

Since tutors of carrier subjects are required to teach the topics of HIV and gender, their preparedness to address these issues varied considerably. Some tutors had not received any training to prepare them in this respect, while others had attended short workshops. For example, one tutor had attended a three-week course for licensed teachers in which HIV was included; another had attended a seminar organised by an NGO. Although we do not have information on the objective or content of these workshops, they seemed to be aimed at raising awareness and providing basic information. A tutor who attended a workshop told us *'I attended a workshop in Mtwara on HIV and AIDS, we discussed topics about transmission and impact [of the virus]'.*

Two of the six colleges had introduced special classes for teaching HIV. In one college, this had happened after some teachers attended a workshop on family life education and decided to begin holding one session per week to discuss issues related to HIV and gender. However, these sessions did not last long:

> *'We used to have HIV and AIDS education every Monday, where gender and*

HIV and AIDS issues were addressed. But with time students' attendance was not good. We failed to know the reasons; probably students were not interested or they found [the topics] irrelevant'.

(College Principal)

A private university, which also offered certificate and diploma courses, introduced HIV as a separate subject as part of project EDU (*Elimu Dhidi ya Ukimwi* or HIV and AIDS Education). First and second year certificate students attended one 45-minute session per week using materials provided by the project (these materials were not accessible to us). The university also reported organising sessions conducted by medical doctors from a nearby college to talk about HIV. All staff and students of the university were required to attend.

Tutors and trainees in Tanzania reported spending even less time on the topic of gender than on HIV. The responses from the colleges varied, but some students said that they had spent one hour on the topic in two years. In one college, no one mentioned anything about addressing gender-related topics; in another, a tutor mentioned teaching about gender roles through role play; and in a third university college, gender was taught as a separate subject. Some trainees were aware that the topic was to be taught in the development studies course in the diploma programme, but this had not happened at the time of the interviews. Tutors could list what they had taught, such as family relationships, unequal opportunities, biological differences between men and women, and differences in men and women's roles in society, but did not give details of how they taught:

'Regarding gender, I taught the students biological differences between males and females, how roles for both sexes [are] defined in our societies. Some of the roles are for women and some for men. But apart from that I encouraged them to respect each other and work together, and girls to be confident to take some roles and responsibilities like college leadership'.

Only one trainee described how the topic of gender was taught: '*In HIV and AIDS there were discussions and presentations, but in gender it was more teacher-centred lectures*'. At the private university college in our sample, gender studies was offered as a separate subject. Teaching at this university seemed to be more practical and one of the trainees described what they had done during the graduate course:

'We studied gender. We discussed the case of Tanzania by looking at enrolment trends from primary to university level. We realised that as you go to higher levels of education, [the] number of girls decreases as compared to boys. We evidenced this in our college by looking at the students sponsored by the ministry ... We participated in practicum; we visited secondary schools to educate teachers on involvement of students in school activities by considering gender equality'. (Trainee)

Both trainees and tutors seem to view gender education as learning about differences between the sexes or learning about gender roles in society, and something that is appropriate for girls to know.

'It is good to include gender in home economics, because it will help girl students to be confident in making decisions'. (Tutor)

'I learned that even women can take on roles and responsibilities that can be done by men in different offices and institutions like government offices...'. (Trainee)

'Teachers should teach women their roles without misusing their authority'. (Trainee)

It is apparent that the concept of gender education is narrowly defined, and since it is integrated into other subjects, tutors either exclude the topic or approach it from the perspective of those subjects such as biology, where the biological differences between male and female are the focus, or development studies, where they may lecture on what role women can take in development or in their families. Gender issues seem to be understood and represented as women's 'issues', and there was some resentment of this among male trainees:

'There is a need to have fair treatment in advocating gender, because some organisations advocate women's empowerment to the extent of suppressing and humiliating men'. (Trainee)

'Gender equity should be addressed in the right way, because trends show that men are victims of the move'. (Trainee)

Neither the syllabus nor the tutors provide any input on how teachers could optimise learning opportunities for both girls and boys in schools and classrooms. At least one trainee suggested that this was needed: *'There is [a] need to reinforce gender education in our schools. We need tutors to teach us how to bring gender balance in our schools'*. None of the tutors interviewed across all the colleges reported attending any training, workshops or seminars on gender education.

Trainees and tutors interviewed reported that internal tests (conducted by the college or university) and examinations (conducted by the ministry) in some subjects such as development studies and civics include one question on HIV. Despite considerable efforts, we could not access copies of final examination papers for certificates or diplomas. However, we did find a mock examination paper, developed by one of the colleges in our sample, for a general studies course (later renamed development studies) for a single year, 2006. The paper contained 16 questions in the paper, nine of which were compulsory. One of these was on HIV, and asked students to identify the difference between HIV and AIDS. A second was on gender, and required students to identify the gender gap in Tanzania. Both questions attempted to check basic knowledge about the topics. Of the seven optional questions, one required students to discuss the importance of women's empowerment in controlling the spread of STDs and HIV. This single sample of examination question suggests that trainees are tested on basic knowledge about the topics, at least in one of the courses. In general, tutors repeatedly said that trainees give importance to topics that are necessary to learn in order to pass examinations, and that HIV and gender are not significant to passing the certificate or diploma exam.

In Tanzania, the implementation of the curriculum varies across subjects and training colleges. It seems that in most colleges the topic of HIV is taught in science and biology, but very little time is spent on this in other subjects. The main gap between the syllabi and implementation is in the use of participatory teaching methodology, which is recommended but not appropriately implemented. Discussions and group work are primarily used for traditional purposes of requiring students to answer questions asked by the text or the tutor. Another gap between the syllabi and practice is the lack of teaching and learning materials in colleges. The syllabi recommend using a variety of materials (including visual material), but the tutors and colleges have minimal materials available to them. Thus, lack of materials and tutors' poor preparation for providing HIV and gender education within the traditional and religious context of Tanzania are two problems that negatively influence the integration of HIV and gender in practice.

Uganda

HIV and gender are taught both at primary teachers' colleges and at the university in Uganda; however, the emphasis and time spent on these topics varies. When asked about how much time was spent on teaching these topics in class, both tutors and teacher trainees found it extremely hard to quantify. There was no consensus on this, but it was generally agreed that mention of HIV is made at least every week, nearly always through assembly messages and topic integration in various other subjects. It was even more difficult to quantify time spent on gender-related topics, because gender lacks the visibility of HIV:

> *'I have told you there is no specific time for gender and HIV and AIDS ... they appear within other topics. They appear and we teach them. They are not so frequent that we teach them once a week ... maybe fortnightly'.* (Tutor)

As already described in the last chapter and tables 7.6 and 7.7, HIV and gender are rarely mentioned in curriculum documents. However, these topics are hosted in science with health education, professional studies and cultural education. In science, the topic is taught as a 'reproductive health and sex education' issue. Tutors of science, English and professional education studies described how they had dealt with the topic in class:

> *'We discussed the history of HIV: What is HIV? What is AIDS? I taught prevention of HIV, where I explained how to use a male condom theoretically because I did not have a condom to use as a teaching aid. But I explained everything, how to put it on, how to remove it and check for [the] expiry date'.*

> *'I taught HIV and AIDS during [a] debate. The motion was whether men or women spread HIV more than the other. Men won the motion, because the women were few and ladies are not assertive; they could not argue and give facts. For example, men are polygamous so they can bring HIV from the women he goes out with. We also had another motion on whether war or HIV has killed more people?'*

> *'I taught HIV and AIDS while we were discussing life skills. We discussed how one can stay safe by knowing more about relationships. One should know those who are infected and therefore know how to relate with them. S/he should not have [a] sexual relationship with them'.*

As can be seen in the above quotes, tutors attempt to use participatory approaches such as discussion and debate; however, they are unable to use it effectively. For example, in the second quote the tutor is unable to deal with the highly gendered and negative outcome of the debate, or appreciate the false learning and attitudes the debate and its conclusion would have endorsed.

As the following quotes from trainees suggest, a teacher's inability to use participatory methods or to use real materials effectively, lack of textbooks and large classrooms are some of the factors influencing the teaching of HIV, and most probably other subjects.

> *'These sessions [on HIV and AIDS] are lecture-based and sometimes teacher-lead discussions. The teacher asks questions and we respond. We also had a session in which we discussed transmission, in which the teacher brought razor blades and syringes as examples of sharp objects which can transmit HIV if shared. Each table had these resources per three students'.*

> *'The textbooks are not enough; we share one book between three students. We need other resources for teaching and learning. We need charts and audio-visual materials. There were no teaching aids like male and female condoms'.*

> *'We are also too many in our class for effective learning: 80 trainees in one stream and 60 in the other stream'.*

HIV inclusion and coverage of content varies across the teaching of courses and, as one tutor stated, '*tutors are expected to integrate it [HIV] where it is applicable*'. Another tutor explained this further:

> *'HIV and AIDS is included in the science syllabus. In the other subjects, teachers are supposed to integrate it. For example, in English language, they can include it in debates and comprehension passages. In music, dance and drama, they can compose songs and perform skits on HIV themes. In [the] foundation of education subject, a tutor can integrate HIV and AIDS education when teaching life skills. But in all these subjects, HIV education is not stated as a topic or a subtopic. Although HIV is not included in the other subjects apart from science, we tutors are expected [by the college] to integrate it in our lessons where it can fit. We also talk about HIV during school assemblies. The messages are usually meant for awareness. We tell them not to engage in sexual activities because they can get HIV'.*

With integration being left to the discretion of individual tutors, each tutor uses a different approach. However, common features in the approaches are awareness and sensitisation messages, as reported by a music tutor:

> *'I integrate HIV/gender in the music components I teach. In PIASCY reform activities HIV forms a focal point, as most themes for the competitions to be staged are on HIV; you can say that some dances are for girls, others are for boys. Culturally, there are courtship dances for each gender. But the topic is not coming out clearly. In the process of teaching, we mix them, e.g. Rakar-aka [a local traditional dance from Northern Uganda] was meant for girls to be admired by men. We don't have a separate course for HIV/gender'.*

Tutors and trainees in Uganda reported that awareness messages and information are delivered during assemblies, through clubs, e.g. the Family Life Club, public lectures and presentations by resource persons from various non-governmental organisations involved in HIV and gender activities, the Health Department, youth organisations, religious organisations, such as the Catholic Church and Uganda Muslim Supreme Council, and the Human Rights Commission. However, we could not confirm this through observation.

Many tutors and students interviewed referred to materials developed by the Presidential Initiative on the AIDS Strategy for Communication to Youth (PIASCY) UPHOLD (Uganda Programme for Human and Holistic Development), REPLICA (Revitalisation of Education, Participation and Learning in Conflict Areas) and FAWE (Forum for African Women Educationists). Even though these materials are not included in the formal PTE curriculum document, the Ministry of Education and Sports (MOES) supports its use in colleges and the university. Some tutors in the sample colleges had been trained on how to use the material by the MOES; this training provides useful skills, knowledge and resources for use in primary schools and teacher education. A tutor who had attended the training said *'It [PIASCY material] is the main book we use … it would be difficult to handle the subject [HIV] during practice teaching without it [PIASCY material]'*.

Even though these materials were available in all colleges in our sample, their use varied. In three colleges, the material was available in the library and there was evidence of use in the classroom and in assemblies. In one college, the material was stored in the one of the administrator's offices and not used. Because PIASCY material is not in the mainstream college curriculum, tutors and students may choose to use it or not.

Although some HIV education is being provided at Uganda's primary teachers' colleges (PTCs), both tutors and principals strongly expressed the desire that HIV teaching should be mainstreamed into the formal primary teacher education curriculum:

> *'Let HIV education be included in the curriculum as an independent subject because there is too much content to be taught within the limitations of the present curriculum. As a teacher going to the field, I'm going to carry out vocational and social education and guidance and counselling'.*
>
> (PTC tutor)

They argued that the teaching, learning and assessment of HIV would be more effective if it was integrated as a stand-alone subject within the curriculum, or as a clearly specified examinable topic area in particular subjects – so that teaching is not left to the discretion of the tutor. The management of the HIV curriculum in its current state was further described as *'a vision that is short term'*. According to both tutors and teacher trainees, the current prescribed curriculum for primary teacher education lacks books and material for teaching HIV and AIDS. Trainees complained that the teaching of HIV had the same focus at all levels of education, leading to message fatigue. As the head of department, teacher education, at the university observed *'there is [a] need to move HIV and AIDS from the A (abstinence) B (be faithful) and C (condomise) to "D" to "Z"'*.

The integration and teaching of gender education in Uganda is even less than for HIV. Tutors and teacher trainees are limited in their understanding of gender, because gender in primary teacher education is taught as sex roles. Even though there is an attempt to raise awareness of gender equity and equality, 'sex roles' is approached from a social and cultural point of view, where teacher trainees are taught that girls 'should cook' and 'be disciplined' while boys should 'care for the home' and 'look after cattle'. For a topic area that should equip future teachers with the knowledge and skills necessary to deal with negative social and cultural attitudes towards gender, this current approach fails to sufficiently challenge social and cultural definitions of gender. In addition, this approach is not a particularly good gender responsive pedagogy for use among teacher trainees.

Teaching and learning materials and training on gender responsive pedagogy is provided by FAWE (Mlama et al., 2005; REPLICA, 2006). In the sample for this study, only one tutor had received training and reported he practiced this in his class. However, most tutors said that they lacked awareness of gender responsive pedagogy. This, along with the absence of gender-related objectives and content in the curriculum, may explain gender education as it is offered in the colleges. According to one student '*gender should be taught, it has not been taken seriously*', and according to tutors, teaching on gender is on the whole '*confusing*' because '*people jump to sex*'.

At the university, the teaching of HIV and gender education depends on the interest and capacity of the tutors. Most tutors felt that the HIV and gender content included in degree programmes for teachers was inadequate. Seven out of the ten lecturers interviewed reported taking personal initiatives to integrate HIV education into their teaching occasionally and when there was a prompting opportunity. In doing so, they mostly provide messages of caution and awareness. Three of the ten spend time on topics related to HIV and gender to teach awareness, control and prevention, as well as to cover subject-specific content, which includes facts and sensitisation information related particularly to HIV and AIDS.

> '*I want boys and girls to be empowered so that they don't catch the disease. I emphasise the ABC (which focuses on the avoidance of HIV), whenever it is appropriate and necessary during my teaching. There is no programme, but a proposal was written to ask for support*'. (University lecturer)

> '*I handle HIV informally as a "by-the-way"; i.e. out of concern I give cautions and guidance where necessary. I have not taught gender/HIV education deliberately*'. (University lecturer)

The lack of specified course content means that teaching is erratic, as a BEd student reported:

> '*We have not yet studied any sessions on HIV and gender, but we hope to study it this academic year under professional studies (PS) according to the course outline. In religious studies (RS) we study gender roles under ethics, but HIV is not projected anywhere in religious studies. HIV content is found in professional studies [and] ECED under health education*'.

Another student explained the sessions on gender within religious studies. These sessions seem to endorse preordained gender roles and do not encourage questioning or changing those roles:

> *'The sessions we covered in religious studies were useful in that they highlighted our responsibilities, i.e. men and women as co-creators; we understood our respective contribution and [the] need to work together complementarily. We also examined the impact of culture on the leadership roles of women, but we found that the Biblical scriptures give a controversial perspective, where some sacraments are only for men like ordination. Also in The Bible, language is still exclusive; some religious scriptures depict that women's role is slightly above that of a slave. Women need to take up positions for empowerment, educating teachers to treat children fairly'.*

While students report learning from session on HIV and gender, they also suggested that the teaching was sometimes ineffective. For example, some male students complained that gender education was delivered as a 'women's' issue and aggravated male students enough for them to lose interest: *'gender is projected in a biased way, so we [men] switch off, but culture still pulls women down'.*

With regard to HIV, many Ugandan youth have grown up with HIV messages around them. By the time they are in university, there is fatigue towards the topic. The remarks below capture the apathy among students, and the need for university lecturers to find creative ways of teaching the HIV curriculum.

> *'To many students, especially girls, HIV seems not to be a sensitive thing. They see it as fun; they make fun out of the caution and advice given, say about the vulnerability of females. Students think the risk is further from them. They don't take it serious[ly]'.*

> *'The BEd students seem to take issues discussed seriously, because they are mature and have adolescent children back home. The BA (Education) students are reluctant to discuss HIV and gender issues and seem bored and tormented by the daily song on HIV and AIDS'.*

> *'We need real materials, e.g. condoms, because there are some students who have never seen condoms. [We] also [need] resource persons, Straight Talk*

and Youth Alive books [materials on reproductive health for young people focussing on behaviour change], novels [and] videos'.

While the country's curriculum and college management expect tutors to translate and enrich the curriculum in their practice, many tutors feel that they do not have preparation enough to do so. Generally, tutors reported that the teaching of HIV is no longer embarrassing. However, they also claimed that teaching materials were inadequate and that they lacked the knowledge necessary to prepare good teachers:

'If someone comes to you and sees knowledge, before even talking to you [they] say, "That one is a teacher. That one is special". But, how can you be special when you lack knowledge to counsel and guide? It is [up to] teachers to teach both parents and students'.

This responsibility is perceived in a much broader sense as holding knowledge for the community. Such a role is possible where teaching and learning resources are improved *'let the government equip the school with all the teacher needs, so that he [or she] can teach the community ... the teacher is the answer to community'.*

HIV and gender education are not examined consistently, because they are not stand-alone subjects. As a tutor pointed out

'If you look at past papers, very little is examined on HIV, meaning therefore it does not give students a sense that it is very important'.

HIV-related knowledge is assessed through class tests in science, but these tests are primarily about basic knowledge, e.g. definitions, causes, transmission and preventative measures. How teachers will use this knowledge to teach in their classes may be assessed during school practice:

'We assess through supervision of school practice (SP) to see how PIASCY knowledge and skills are utilised during teaching – we look at how the students use or integrate HIV messages in the compound or in the classroom during teaching. Treatment given to sick children and utterances made by trainees are watched keenly. Some questions on HIV come [up] in the test or examination in science, but not frequently of course'.

The majority of tutors and teacher trainees in Uganda believe that formal assessment of HIV and gender education would help the subject to be taken more seriously. One tutor accurately captured the sentiments of the others: '*Specific topics stipulated for gender and HIV and AIDS should be examined, because people are examination oriented in Uganda*'. The university lecturers felt that more practical assessment is required, so that students acquire the skills and understanding of what does and does not work in real situations.

Like the other two countries, there is a gap between curriculum documents and actual practice in pre-service teacher education in Uganda. The curriculum has not been reviewed in some years, and hence does not integrate HIV education as explicitly as the curricula in the other two countries.

Chapter 9

Gaps Between Policy, Curriculum and Practice Across the Three Countries

The three countries in our review have a strong and encouraging policy context, and this encourages and indeed mandates the inclusion of HIV and AIDS education into the school curricula and by extension into teacher training. However, the gap between policy and implementation is wide. Although most training in HIV education for teachers is short and takes place in-service, the three countries have included HIV education in their school curricula. It is integrated or infused into the curricula of certificate, diploma and degree courses for teacher preparation. Science, social studies, civics and religious and development studies seem to be the main carrier subjects. However, the objectives and the content on HIV and gender aim only at providing factual knowledge and raising awareness among teachers. They do not reflect the aim of preparing future teachers to teach children and young adults to change their behaviour.

Teacher education colleges across the three countries intend to integrate HIV and gender in their teaching. However, teaching on the issues is not systematic and little class time is spent on them. The main focus of HIV teaching is the transmission of scientific and factual knowledge. Little attention is given to engage trainees in examining their existing beliefs, attitudes and behaviours or in learning how to teach these topics to children in schools. Teaching learning materials have been developed in the three countries. However, these are of varying quality, not uniformly available or readily accessible by tutors and trainees and are seldom used in teaching. Moreover, such materials are not prepared to enrich and support the pre-service curricula.

Curricula in the three countries recommend use of participatory teaching approaches in teacher education programmes. However, it is clear that tutors lack adequate preparation to use these approaches effectively themselves or to help prepare future teachers to use them in their school classrooms.

Lack of good teaching learning materials, poor tutor preparation and tutors' lack of ability and interest to integrate HIV and/or gender into the teaching of other subjects are the main reasons for the limited and superficial teaching of these topics in pre-service teacher education. The addition of HIV and gender to other subjects, and the ensuing possibility that the subjects can then be passed without teaching or assessing students on these topics, also conveys the message that HIV and gender are insignificant and non-serious topics and that they are inessential to teacher preparation. Where gender topics are included, they represent a reinforcement of current gender roles and relationships, or take a welfare approach. The curriculum does not include the objective of strengthening women's agency necessary for their wellbeing (Sen, 1999). Gender finds even less space than HIV and AIDS in the curricula and in teaching.

Chapter 10

Recommendations

A general conclusion from this review is that syllabus content, teaching materials and teaching practice in teacher education are inadequate to impact personal beliefs, attitudes and behaviours of future teachers significantly or to prepare them to influence and shape the beliefs, attitudes and behaviours of children and youth in schools about and towards HIV and gender. The syllabus and its implementation in the colleges seem to focus on raising awareness and reviewing trainees' existing knowledge about modes of transmission and prevention, without going into depth. Perhaps there is an assumption that this awareness will lead to changes in behaviour. That this is an unwarranted assumption is underscored by the recommendations presented below. These emanate from our review and from the suggestions made by tutors and trainees in the colleges in our sample.

1. HIV and AIDS education should be a separate examinable subject. This would increase its importance for both tutors and trainee teachers, provide adequate time to deal with the topic in depth and ensure equal opportunities for all trainees. Currently, those who take biology or civics receive more input than those with different specialisations. However, if this is impossible to do in an already crowded curriculum, there should be a more thoughtful integration across the existing course.

2. A variety of teaching learning materials to support pre-service teacher education, with better content relevant to HIV and gender education, should be available at all teacher training colleges. At present, syllabi recommend that tutors use a variety of materials, including video. However, such materials are unavailable in the colleges, and tutors depend on information that students might already have or on other sources such as subject modules or course books for basic science subjects.

3. Curricula should include the objective of developing teachers' knowledge and ability to provide HIV and AIDS education to children in schools. Existing curricula completely ignore this aspect.

4. Tutors themselves need preparation and support to teach these topics to future teachers. Professional development programmes must be organised to support tutors to become effective teacher educators, who can prepare and support teacher trainees to teach HIV and gender education to young people and address related issues in schools.

5. Tutor preparation programmes must include opportunities for teacher educators and teachers to examine and challenge their own existing beliefs and attitudes about HIV and gender.

6. At present, curricula recommend participatory methods, but tutors are unable to implement those methods effectively. Tutors need a clear understanding of the purpose of participatory methods, and a better ability to use them effectively. Professional development for tutors and pre-service courses for teachers must ensure that this need is addressed.

7. While tutors and trainees express awareness of the significance of HIV education for all, they lack similar awareness of the relevance of gender to the process of teaching and learning. Gender education for teachers must emphasise examination of their own concepts and beliefs about gender and understanding of a teacher's responsibility to practice gender-aware pedagogy.

8. Teacher education curricula should adequately address the need to prepare teachers to be aware of gender inequality, to promote gender equality and to adopt gender-sensitive pedagogy in their own practices. Curricula must also highlight the links between gender and HIV and AIDS.

Appendix

HIV and AIDS and Gender Study Dissemination Workshop, 11–13 March 2008

A three-day workshop was held to share initial findings from the curriculum review, to obtain responses from stakeholders, to broaden our understanding of the issues around HIV and AIDS and gender in teacher education, and to obtain participants' recommendations on how to improve the curriculum and its implementation. Representatives from the Ministry of Education in the three countries, principals and a tutor from each of the colleges in the sample attended the workshop. Here we summarise the workshop discussion.

There are common themes threading through the teacher education practices of the three countries, and several common issues arise in regard to HIV and gender in teacher education:

- Teacher educators, teachers and the community have rigid attitudes
- Media: how can education influence the media?
- Cultural context: beliefs and biases negatively contribute to the spread of HIV
- Dissemination of contradictory information by different bodies (the media, churches, schools)
- HIV is impacting negatively on education, because the teachers who are seen as key persons in disseminating information are most affected by HIV and AIDS
- Gaps in ministry of education policies and PTCs
- Mismatch in primary and PTC curricula

Gender and HIV are interlinked. HIV and AIDS prevalence is higher in women of productive age groups; so we need to empower women/girls to value themselves – women can play an important role in the reduction of HIV infection if they understand their worth. At the same time, education is expected to address the HIV and AIDS epidemic; so we need to find workable solutions to change the mindset of our society, using friendly means.

The education sectors in all three countries have yet to make satisfactory interventions regarding HIV in teacher education. The issue of HIV has not been mainstreamed in the various curricula of teacher education across the three countries: HIV is taught as a topic in science in some institutions, but in most teacher education institutions it is only infused. Such integration is not carried out clearly; most curricula have no content on HIV and AIDS.

Teaching HIV education is theoretical and generally haphazard (informal); hence youths and many other people have reasonable knowledge about HIV and AIDS, but lack the skills and attitudes to apply that knowledge. To create any impact, the curricula must target attitudinal change. Nor is assessment performed effectively, as it involves a lot of 'knowledge questions'.

NGOs have spearheaded sensitisation on HIV and AIDS in primary schools, but content has not been reflected in the formal curricula. Once projects close, then the initiative dies. Teacher educators admitted that they are not competent in dealing with HIV and gender education. They need training in methodology to be able to teach HIV and AIDS with expertise.

In terms of differences, Tanzania has a policy, but implementation needs improvement. Uganda, meanwhile, has made many interventions, but these have been through NGOs and sustainability is a big issue.

Way forward

Participants engaged in constructive and open discussions around several questions. Key ideas generated from the discussion were:

- What kind of teachers do we want?
  Gender and HIV conscious and competent; diversified and comprehensive enough to integrate cultural and religious values with scientific knowledge

- What type of syllabus/curriculum (content) do we need to bring about positive change?
  Holistic, dynamic and gender responsive and HIV alert

- What methods will be most effective?
  (Experiential and participatory)
- What outcomes do we expect?
  Individuals all round being endowed with the necessary life skills to live and survive in the era of HIV and AIDS
  Participants noted that:
- There is a great challenge ahead of us, to effectively package the content of HIV and AIDS and gender if it is to be acceptable to the different stakeholders in education.
- The type of content for teacher educators and how it should be delivered need to be well thought out to make lessons practical and meaningful for attitudinal change
- We need to concert efforts as East Africans, share information and develop teaching materials that will be user-friendly, but also provide an effective means of creating impact. Students need vibrant approaches, because they are bored of the same threats that accompany lessons on HIV and AIDS.
- Students prefer videos about HIV and AIDS affected/infected persons to give real experiences.
- Life skills education is crucial in the fight against HIV, as it will empower children, youths and adults to make informed choices.
- Above all, we need to handle all current issues and challenges with sensitivity to multiple cultural biases.
- Training teachers is essential to enable them to develop confidence – to create a learner-friendly environment, and to deliver content on HIV through participatory methods, which tend to be more popular.
- Key challenges: teacher institutions are ill-resourced, time is scarce due to the competing programmes hosted in training institutions, and curricula of both schools and training institutions are already fatigued.

Notes

1 HIV: Human immunodeficiency virus, a retro-virus which causes AIDS. AIDS: Acquired immune deficiency syndrome.
2 Some countries, such as Tanzania, have introduced one year at teacher training college followed by a year of deployment in schools so as to learn 'in the field'.
3 The gross enrolment rate is the number of students enrolled at a certain level of education regardless of age as a percentage of the population of official school age.
4 Teacher Training College.
5 National Training College.
6 This is probably a reference to female genital mutilation.
7 Each school subject area has an academic and a pedagogy syllabus. So, for example, biology has a biology academic syllabus and biology pedagogy syllabus.

References

Bennell, P and Mukyanuzi, F (2005). 'Is there a teacher motivation crisis in Tanzania?', retrieved 2 December 2008 from: www.eldis.org/vfile/upload/1/document/0709/Teacher_motivation_Tanzania.pdf

Clarke, D (2005). 'Planning and evaluation for gender equality in education in the context of HIV and AIDS', retrieved 2 December 2008 from: http://www.ungei.org/resources/1612_614.html

Cohen, D (2002). 'Human capital and the HIV epidemic in sub-Saharan Africa', Working Paper 2, Geneva: ILO Program on AIDS and the World Bank.

Colclough, C, Al-Samaari, S, Rose, P and Tembon, M (2003). *Achieving Schooling for All in Africa: Costs, Constraints and Gender*. Aldershot: Ashgate Publishing Limited.

Darling-Hammond, L (2000). 'Teacher Quality and Student Achievement: A Review of State Policy', *Educational Policy Analysis Archives*, 8 (1).

Government of Kenya, Ministry of Health (2008). See: www.health.go.ke/ (accessed 13 June 2000).

Government of Uganda (1992). *Government White Paper on the Education Policy Review Commission Report*. Kampala: Government Printers.

Government of Uganda (2001). 'Education in Uganda in the Last Ten Years', A paper presented at International Conference on Education, Geneva, 5–7 September 2001.

Government of Uganda (2003). *Laws of Uganda 2000*, chapter 59: 'The Children Act'. Kampala: Government Printers.

Government of Uganda (2004). *The National Orphans and Other Vulnerable Children Policy*. Kampala: Government Printers.

Government of Uganda (2005). *Follow-up to the Declaration of Commitment on HIV and AIDS*. Kampala: Uganda AIDS Commission.

Government of Uganda (2006). *The Education Sector HIV and AIDS Workplace Policy*. Kampala: Government Printers.

Hargreaves J and Boler, T (2006). 'Girl Power: the Impact of Girls' Education on HIV and Sexual Behaviour'. Johannesburg: Action Aid International. Accessed 20 May 2008 from: www.oxfamkic.org

James-Traore, TA, Finger, W, Ruland, CD and Savariaud, S (2004). 'Teacher Training: Essential for School-based Reproductive Health and HIV/AIDS

Education. Focus on Sub-Saharan Africa'. Arlington, Virginia: Family Health International (FHI), YouthNet (Youth Issues Paper No.3).

Joint UN Programme on HIV/AIDS (UNAIDS) (2008a). *2007 Sub-Saharan Africa. AIDS Epidemic Update: Regional Summary*. Accessed 15 June 2008 from: data.unaids.org/pub/Report/2008/jc1526_epibriefs_ssafrica_en.pdf

Joint UN Programme on HIV/AIDS (UNAIDS) (2008b). *Report on the Global AIDS Epidemic*. Accessed 15 June 2008 from: www.unaids.org/en/Knowledge Centre/HIVData/GlobalReport/2008_global_report.asp

Kakuru, DM (2007). Gender Equality and HIV and AIDS in Uganda. In *id Insights: Research Findings for Development Policymakers and Practitioners*. Brighton: Institute of Development Studies, University of Sussex.

Kawewa, J (undated). *Situational Analysis on HIV AND AIDS in Kenya*. Department of Adult Education. Retrieved 19 June 2008, from: http://www.unesco.org/education/uie/pdf/Kawewa.pdf

Lewin, KM (2003). 'Some Teacher Training Issues in Tanzania: Projecting Supply and Demand', Briefing paper presented at a conference in Arusha, Tanzania, December 2003. Government of Tanzania and World Bank 2003/4.

Lindhe, V, Malmberg, K and Temu, BE (2005). *Sida Support to Teacher Education in Tanzania 1997–2002*. Sida Evaluation 05/05. Stockholm: Swedish International Development Cooperation Agency.

Ministry of Education (1995). *Tanzania Education and Training Policy*. Government of Tanzania.

Ministry of Education and Sports (MOES) (1994). *Syllabus for primary teachers' colleges*. Kampala: MOES.

Ministry of Education and Sports, Presidential Initiative on AIDS Strategy for Communication to Youth (PIASCY) (2004). *Helping Pupils to Stay Safe: A Handbook for Teachers*, pp.3–7. Kampala: MOES.

Ministry of Education and Sports (2005). *Education Sector Annual Performance Report*. Retrieved 27 April 2006 from: http://www.education.go.ug/Final%20ESAPR2005.htm

Ministry of Education and Sports (2006a). *Education Sector Annual Performance Report*. Kampala: Government Printers.

Ministry of Education and Sports (2006b). *Uganda Education Statistics Abstract*. Kampala: Government Printers

Ministry of Education, Science and Technology (MOEST) (2004). *Primary Teacher Education Syllabus (Vols 1 and 2)*. Nairobi: Kenya Institute of Education.

Ministry of Education, Science and Technology (2005a). 'A Policy Framework for Education: Training and Research'. Sessional Paper No.1 of 2005. Nairobi: Government Printers.

Ministry of Education, Science and Technology (2005b). *Kenya Education Sector Support Programme 2005–2010: Delivering Quality Education and Training to all Kenyans*. Nairobi: Government Printers.

Ministry of Gender, Sports, Culture and Social Services (MGSC&SS) (2000). *National Gender and Development Policy*. Nairobi: Ministry of Gender, Sports, Culture and Social Services.

Ministry of Science, Technology and Higher Education, United Republic of Tanzania (1999). *National Higher Education Policy*. Dar es Salaam, February 1999. Retrieved May 2007 from: http://www.tanzania.go.tz/pdf/national highereducationpolicy.pdf

Mirembe, R and Davies, L (2001). 'Is Schooling a Risk? Gender, Power Relations and School Culture in Uganda'. In *Gender and Education*, Vol. 13, No.4, pp. 401–416.

Mlama, P, Marema, D and Makoye, H (2005). *Gender Responsive Pedagogy: A Teacher's Handbook*. Nairobi: Forum for African Women Educationalists (FAWE).

National Council for Higher Education (NCHE) (2006). *The State of Higher Education in Uganda*. Kampala: NCHE.

National Institute of Education (2008). *Transforming Teacher Education: Redefined Professionals for 21st Century Schools*. Singapore: Nanyang Technological University.

Owino, PO (2004). *Study of African Universities' Response to HIV and AIDS: Case of Kenya*. Retrieved 10 April 2008 from: http://education clearinghouse.nairobi-unesco.org/docs/Kenya_HIV_AIDS_survey_report_Dr_Philip_Owino.pdf

Population Reference Bureau (PRB) (2008). See: http://www.prb.org/Datafinder/Geography/Summary.aspx?region=48&region_type=2 [accessed 12 August 2008]

Republic of Kenya (ROK) (1964). *Education Commission: The Report of the National Committee on Education Objectives*. Nairobi: Government Printers.

Republic of Kenya (ROK) (1981). *Report of the Presidential Working Party on the Second University in Kenya*. Nairobi: Government Printers.

Revitalisation of Education, Participation and Learning in Conflict Areas (REPLICA) (2006). *The Basics for Promoting Girls' Education: A Handbook for Guiding Action and Mobilising Support*. Kampala: Instant Printers.

Rispel, L, with Letlape, L and Metcalf, C (2006). *Education Sector Responses to*

HIV and AIDS: Learning from Good Practices in Africa. Based on background paper prepared for and the proceedings of the African regional workshop organised jointly by the Commonwealth Secretariat and ADEA and hosted by Human Sciences Research Council on 12–14 September 2006 in Johannesburg, South Africa.

Sen, A (1999). *Development as Freedom*. Oxford: Oxford University Press.

Suleman, S and Rajani, R (2006). *Secondary Education in Tanzania: Key Policy Challenges*. HakiElimu (Tanzania Education and Democracy Organisation) Working Paper Series No. 4.

Tanzanian Population and Development website. See: http://www.angelfire.com/tn/ppu/ [accessed 20 July 2008]

UN Children's Fund (2004). *The State of the World's Children*. Accessed on 29 May 2008 from: http://www.unicef.org/sowc04/sowc04_contents.html

United Nations Development Programme (UNDP) (2007). *2007/2008 Human Development Report, Tanzania*. Retrieved 14 July 2008 from: http://hdrstats.undp.org/countries/country_fact_sheets/cty_fs_TZA.html

United Nations Educational, Scientific and Cultural Organization (UNESCO) Institute of Statistics. See: http://stats.uis.unesco.org/unesco/TableViewer/document.aspx?ReportId=121&IF_Language=eng&BR_Country=7620 (accessed 13 May 2008).

UNESCO (2004). *Education for All Global Monitoring Report 2003/4. Gender and Education for All, the Leap to Equality*. Retrieved 28 May 2008 from: http://portal.unesco.org/education/en/ev.php-URL_ID=23023&URL_DO=DO_TOPIC&URL_SECTION=201.html

UNESCO (2006). *HIV and AIDS Education: Teacher Training and Teaching. A web-based desk study of 10 African countries*. Retrieved 5 June 2008 from: http://portal.unesco.org/education/en/ev.php-URL_ID=47350&URL_DO=DO_TOPIC&URL_SECTION=201.html

UNESCO (2007a). *Education for All Global Monitoring Report 2008. Education for All by 2015, Will We Make It?* Retrieved 28 May 2008 from: http://www.unesco.org/en/education/efareport/reports/2008-mid-term-review/

UNESCO (2007b). *UNESCO Country Programming Document for the United Republic of Tanzania, 2008–2010*. Paris: UNESCO.

UNGASS (2008a). *United Nations General Assembly Special Session on HIV and AIDS. Country Report – Kenya*. Retrieved 12 June 2008 from: data.unaids.org/pub/Report/2008/Kenya_2008_country_progress_report_en.pdf

UNGASS (2008b). UNGASS Country Progress Report Tanzania Mainland

Jan 2006–Dec 2007. Retrieved 12 June 2008 from: data.unaids.orgs/pub/Report/2008/Tanzania_2008_country_progress_report_en.pdf

Vavrus, F (2003). *Desire and Decline: Schooling Amid Crisis in Tanzania.* Peter Lang Publishing.

Wepukhulu, B (2002). *Capacity Building for Lead Teacher Training Institutions in Tanzania.* Report Submitted to UNESCO headquarters. Paris: UNESCO.

Woods, E (2007). 'Education for All by 2015: Will We Make It? Tanzania country case study'. Background paper for EFA Global Monitoring Report 2008.

World Bank Group (2008). World Development Indicators database, April 2008. Retrieved 28 June 2008 from:

http://ddpext.worldbank.org/ext/ddpreports/ViewSharedReport?&CF=&REPORT_ID=9147&REQUEST_TYPE=VIEWADVANCED&HF=N/CPProfile.asp&WSP=N